# Maternity Nursing

Third Edition

## nursing outline series

D1453898

**Arlyne Friesner, Ed.D., R.N.**
*Dean,* School of Nursing
College of New Rochelle
New Rochelle, New York

**Beverly Raff, Ph.D., R.N.**
*Vice President,* Professional Education
March of Dimes Birth Defects Foundation
White Plains, New York

**Medical Examination Publishing Co., Inc.**
*an Excerpta Medica company*

Friesner, Arlyne.
   Maternity nursing.

   (Nursing outline series)
   Bibliography: p.
   Includes index.
   1. Obstetrical nursing. I. Raff, Beverly.
II. Title. III. Series. [DNLM: 1. Obstetrical
nursing--Outlines. WY F9120]
RG951.F76 1982    610.73'678'076        81-14080
ISBN 0-87488-377-6                      AACR2


Copyright © 1982 by
MEDICAL EXAMINATION PUBLISHING CO., INC.
an Excerpta Medica company
969 Stewart Avenue
Garden City, New York

June 1982

To Joe and Lester

# Contents

# Foreword

Maternity teachers, students, and clinicians are faced daily with increasing knowledge in the field of maternity nursing as well as its complex humanistic aspects.

Teachers of maternity nursing have perhaps the most difficult task, for it is they who are responsible for students' mastery of those fundamental concepts and principles which will assure safe practice. Most nursing programs only allocate one semester for maternal child nursing, which includes both maternity nursing and nursing of children, each with its own text of anywhere from 1,000 to 2,000 pages.

This present edition is thus a welcome teaching resource which does not replace the traditional text, but rather organizes the content so that classroom time can be available for discussion. The teacher who lectures in order to outline basic concepts is using time which could be used more productively in helping students meet the challenges of maternity care - time that could be used for discussion of new developments; for fostering attitudes about moral and ethical issues; and for relating theory to the students' clinical practice.

The authors' questions at the end of each unit, and the sections in many chapters titled "What Remains to be Done," will help the reader to understand the various biological and social forces and developments impinging on the achievement of a more humane and effective delivery of maternity care.

The book's greatest asset is that it provides the reader with a brief, accessible, current, and quick reference guide. As the authors point out, it provides rapid access to the physiological and psychological changes occurring in the maternity cycle and the nursing implications of these changes.

The authors are to be commended for producing this useful and practical volume which can enhance the role of the nurse in maternity so that "the very quality of life itself" may be improved.

M. Elaine Wittmann, Ed.D. , R.N.
Professor of Nursing
Director, Undergraduate Nursing Program
Adelphi University School of Nursing
Garden City, New York

# Preface

The third edition of Maternity Nursing has an updated and expanded text with a particular emphasis on the sections devoted to the high-risk maternity client and preventative prenatal care. The emphasis in this third edition on client's rights and client advocacy remain an essential part of the author's philosophy of nursing care.

The role of the maternity nurse includes involvement in all of the levels of health care; preventative, curative and rehabilitative. In order to deliver this kind of comprehensive health care, the nurse needs precise knowledge of the physiological and psychological changes occurring during the maternity cycle and an awareness of the influence of biophysical and psychosocial environmental factors on the health status and needs of the childbearing family.

The goal of this book is to provide essential knowledge needed by maternity nurses in a concise outline format. The outline format should prove helpful to student nurses who are preparing for State Board Examinations and College Proficiency Examinations. The text is also useful as a study guide to supplement a regular textbook for students who are enrolled in maternity nursing courses. The compact nature of the book makes it a useful reference manual for graduate practicing maternity nurses.

# Acknowledgments

We wish to acknowledge, with sincere gratitude, the technical assistance of Julie Friesner and Rose Stein, and Nancy Schwarzkopf for the illustrations which she contributed.

## notice

The authors and the publisher of this book have made every effort to ensure that all therapeutic modalities that are recommended are in accordance with accepted standards at the time of publication.

The drugs specified within this book may not have specific approval by the Food and Drug Administration in regard to the indications and dosages that are recommended by the authors. The manufacturer's package insert is the best source of current prescribing information.

UNIT I:  HISTORY AND TRENDS IN MATERNAL CARE


CHAPTER 1

HISTORICAL PERSPECTIVES


I.   HISTORICAL BACKGROUND

A.   Early tribes of American Indians and African natives
   1. birth process relatively free of complications due to lack
      of disproportion between fetal head and maternal pelvis,
      because inter-tribal marriages were rare
      a) major complications were abnormal presentations
   2. at time of birth, mother usually delivered child herself un-
      less difficulty was encountered and she needed assistance
      of another woman
   3. as time progressed, those women who had experience in
      assisting others gradually became known as midwives
      a) all knowledge of midwifery was based on experience
   4. if midwives were unable to delivery baby, medicine men
      and priests were called in to help through prayer
   5. childbirth associated with mystery and superstition
      a) usually celebrated with some kind of ceremony which
         gave thanks to the gods, or warded off evil spirits
   6. most nomadic groups seemed to have less concern for the
      pregnant woman than more settled groups
   7. period of recuperation varied
      a) some returned to work immediately
      b) others spent days or weeks recuperating
   8. many groups practiced couvade where the father performs
      the act of childbearing.  This ritual presumably drew away
      evil spirits that might harm mother and baby

B.   Egyptian society
   1. highly organized society
   2. priesthood supervised abnormal deliveries
   3. majority of women delivered with assistance of midwives
   4. obstetric forceps used, and cesarean sections were per-
      formed on dead mothers
   5. descriptions of contraceptive methods found in ancient writ-
      ings
   6. first pregnancy test described.  Women would urinate over
      mixture of wheat and barley seeds mixed with dates and
      sand.  If seeds sprouted the test was positive for preg-
      nancy.  This test may have had some success because of
      hormonal content of urine

C. Greek and Roman cultures
 1. in early Grecian history, obstetrics was involved with religious practices such as fertility rites
 2. Hippocratic period
   a) the beginning of the scientific study and practice of medicine
   b) normal deliveries assisted by midwives under supervision of physicians
   c) abnormal labor handled by physicians
   d) Hippocrates wrote about theory and practice of obstetrics
 3. Soranus of Ephesus was called the Father of Obstetrics because he was the first man to write about obstetrical theory and care
   a) wrote about podalic version
 4. Moschion practiced medicine in Rome
   a) wrote textbook for midwives
   b) improved upon Hippocrates' teachings

D. Hebrew culture
 1. although no medical assistance was given for difficult deliveries, cleanliness and good sanitation were practiced and emotional support was provided by family members

E. Eastern cultures
 1. Hindus practiced an organized system of medicine
   a) Susrata's contribution to the scientific knowledge of obstetrics included
     (1) knowledge of menstruation and gestation
     (2) establishment of prenatal and postnatal care
     (3) management of abnormal labor
     (4) use of forceps, and cesarean section on dead mothers
     (5) use of cleanliness and sanitation

F. Medieval period
 1. lack of progress in obstetrical science and practice
 2. loss of knowledge from previous cultures
 3. in Europe there was a regression to mysticism in medical practice
 4. beginning of hospital and nursing services
   a) usually used only for the poor

G. Renaissance period
 1. establishment of Italian medical schools brought about increased knowledge in obstetrics
   a) Arantius: described pregnant uterus and gestational development
   b) Vesalius: accurately described pelvis
 2. William Harvey: described circulation of the blood and physiology of pregnancy

3. Ambrose Pare: reintroduced the use of podalic version in obstetrics and helped establish first midwifery school in France. He also established obstetrical practice as part of medicine
4. handbook for midwives by Jakob Rueff widely used
5. birthing chairs used for delivery
6. Leonardo da Vinci depicted the true position of the fetus in utero

H. Seventeenth century to nineteenth century
1. 1618: Wittenberg performed first cesarean section on a live mother
2. seventeenth century: Mauriceau referred to puerperal fever
3. Chamberlin family designed obstetrical forceps around 1580, but kept information secret until 1813
4. eighteenth century: Palfyne presented obstetric forceps to French Academy of Medicine
5. eighteenth century brought into vogue the use of male physicians as obstetricians
6. eighteenth century: Smellie measured pelvis to determine eventual course of labor
7. eighteenth century: Hunter contributed to the knowledge of placental anatomy
8. colonial American obstetricians studied under Smellie and Hunter who thereby greatly influenced American obstetrical practice
9. puerperal fever
    a) from seventeenth to nineteenth centuries, puerperal fever reached epidemic proportions
    b) in 1795, Gordon called puerperal fever an infectious disease
    c) in 1843, Oliver Wendell Holmes wrote a paper on the contagiousness of puerperal fever and the medical aseptic techniques useful in combating the disease, causing great controversy over his research because scientific knowledge of the germ theory was not yet established
    d) in 1861, Semmelweis published a paper on the method of transmission of puerperal fever and utilized chloride of lime for hand washing which greatly reduced the mortality rate from the disease
    e) in 1860, Pasteur identified the cause of puerperal fever providing the scientific rationale for the theories of Holmes and Semmelweis
10. in 1853, Simpson introduced chloroform as an anesthetic in obstetrics

I. Twentieth century
1. technological advances
    a) advances in anesthetics and analgesia
    b) discovery and use of antibiotics for infection control

      c) the development and use of blood transfusion
      d) development and use of x-ray to determine cephalo-pelvic disproportion
      e) advances in general medical and surgical knowledge
      f) more accurate collection of vital statistics and methods of epidemiological research have improved
      g) improved environment sanitation and communicable disease control
      h) prenatal diagnosis and treatment
      i) fetal monitoring
      j) sonography and amniocentesis developed
      k) fetal surgery

2. twentieth century - philosophical advances
      a) an important factor in improving the outcome of pregnancy during this century is the generally higher standard of living that prevails. Also, after World War II a change in focus from the person providing the care to the recipient brought about a change in terminology, we no longer speak of obstetrical care but rather of maternity care. This had broadened the scope of care to include prenatal and postnatal care which promotes the general health and well-being not only of the mother and child but that of the entire expanding family
      b) WHO definition of maternity care (WHO Report 1952) "The object of maternity care is to ensure that every expectant and nursing mother maintains good health, learns the art of child care, has a normal delivery, and bears healthy children. Maternity care in the narrower sense consists in the care of the pregnant woman, her safe delivery, her postnatal examination, the care of her newly born infant, and the maintenance of lactation. In the wider sense, it begins much earlier in measures aimed to promote the health and well-being of the young people who are potential parents, and to help them develop the right approach to family life and to the place of the family in the community. It should also include guidance in parent-craft and in problems associated with infertility and family planning"

3. advances in research and knowledge
      a) increased knowledge of the role of nutrition in the maternity cycle
      b) increased number of hospital deliveries with excellent control of infection through improved medical and surgical asepsis and the establishment of hospital standards
      c) increased safety in operative obstetrics
      d) improved education to prepare professional practitioners
      e) introduction of prepared childbirth and family-centered maternity care
      f) increased research and progress in pharmacology
      g) expanding knowledge in the field of genetics
      h) treatment of the fetus in utero

J.   Development of maternity nursing
    1. midwifery - has its roots in ancient society
       a) formal training began in eighteenth century
       b) male physicians not involved in normal pregnancies, labor and delivery
    2. maternity nursing
       a) prior to the concept of family-centered maternity care, nursing care was based on meeting the immediate physical and technological needs of the pregnant woman
       b) today, a growing number of nurses are becoming involved with patient education throughout the maternity cycle
       c) nurses are becoming patient advocates and are assisting parents in their quest to fully participate in childbearing

CHAPTER 2

CURRENT PROBLEMS AND TRENDS

I. MODERN TRENDS

A. Development of maternal-child care in U.S.: there has been
a substantial improvement in the health and welfare of mothers
and children over the past 50 years. This improvement is directly attributed to epidemiological research and the increased
quantity and quality of health services offered. In order to understand the implications of past problems and future needs,
it is essential to be familiar with statistical terms and trends
in maternal and child health
1. definitions of statistical terms - rates are for a calendar
year
a) birth rate: number of births per 1000 total population
b) fertility rate: number of live births per 1000 population
of women between the ages of 15 to 44 years
c) neonatal mortality rate: number of deaths during first 4
weeks of life per 1000 live births
d) fetal mortality rate or stillbirth: one in which any prod-
uct of conception of 20 weeks or more gestational age
dies in utero prior to birth, per 1000 live births
e) perinatal mortality rate: number of deaths of fetuses
and neonates from 20 weeks gestation to the twenty-
eighth day of life, per 1000 live births
f) infant mortality rate: number of deaths of infants under
1 year of age, per 1000 live births
g) maternal mortality rate: number of maternal deaths per
100,000 live births
(1) base recently changed from 10,000 live births to
100,000 live births
2. trends in birth rates
a) 1930: 21.7 live births per 1000 total population
b) 1957: 25.3 live births per 1000 total population
c) 1963: 21.7 live births per 1000 total population
d) 1974: 14.9 live births per 1000 total population
(1) this is the lowest birth rate observed in the U.S.
e) 1978: 15.3 live births per 1000 total population
3. trends in fertility rates
a) the childbearing population comprises a smaller proportion of the total than in previous years

6

   (1) 1936 - 24%
   (2) 1974 - 22%
  b) 1918: 125 live births per 1000 women aged 15-44 years
  c) 1930: 90 live births per 1000 women aged 15-44 years
  d) 1957: 122.7 live births per 1000 women aged 15-44 years
  e) 1973: 69.2 live births per 1000 women aged 15-44 years
  f) 1978: 66.6 live births per 1000 women aged 15-44 years
4. trends in maternal death rates
  a) 1915: 60 maternal deaths per 10,000 live births
  b) 1960: 2.7 maternal deaths per 10,000 live births
  c) 1971: 20.5 maternal deaths per 100,000 live births
  d) 1974: 14.6 maternal deaths per 100,000 live births
  e) 1978: 9.6 maternal deaths per 100,000 live births
   (USPHS 1980)
5. trends in infant death rates
  a) 1915: 100 infant deaths per 1000 live births
  b) 1969: 20.7 infant deaths per 1000 live births
  c) 1971: 19.2 infant deaths per 1000 live births
  d) 1974: 16.7 infant deaths per 1000 live births
  e) 1978: 13.8 infant deaths per 1000 live births (USPHS 1980)
  f) 1979: 13.0 infant deaths per 1000 live births (NAACOG Bull. 1981)
6. significance of statistical trends
  a) the overall statistical facts do not give an accurate picture of the differences in maternal and infant death rates for
   (1) high and low income groups
   (2) white and nonwhite groups
   (3) urban and rural areas
  b) low income groups, nonwhite groups, and those living in rural areas, have a higher maternal and infant death rate than the national average
   (1) infant death rate in U.S. in 1968 was 21.8 per 1000 live births
   (2) racial breakdown of infant death rate for the year 1968
    (a) nonwhite: 34.5 per 1000 live births
    (b) white: 19.2 per 1000 live births
   (3) 1977: infant death rate was 14.1 per 1000 live births
   (4) racial breakdown of infant death rate for the year 1977
    (a) nonwhite: 21.7
    (b) white: 12.3
   (5) maternal mortality rate in U.S. for 1968 was 24.5 per 100,000 live births
   (6) racial breakdown of maternal death rates for the year of 1968
    (a) nonwhite: 63.6 per 100,000 live births
    (b) white: 16.6 per 100,000 live births

    (7) maternal mortality rate in U.S. for 1977 was 11.2 per 100,000 live births

    (8) racial breakdown of maternal death rates for the year 1977
        (a) nonwhite: 26.0 per 100,000 live births
        (b) whites: 7.7 per 100,000 live births

    (9) in 1974 in New York State the infant mortality rate was 16.3 and in Mississippi, a predominantly rural state, it was 23.0

    (10) in 1977 in New York State the infant mortality rate was 13.0 and in Mississippi it was 18.2

    (11) the range of infant mortality in the United States by state in 1979 (NAACOG Bull. 1981)
        (a) low of 10.4 in Maine and New Hampshire
        (b) high of 19.3 in District of Columbia and 14.8 in Mississippi

    (12) neonatal mortality decreased by 39% for blacks between 1965-1974 compared to 46% for whites

7. factors contributing to differences in infant and maternal death rates

  a) low birth weight is the major cause of infant deaths (Surg. Gen. Report 1980)
    (1) low-weight infants (under 5.5 lbs) are 40 times as likely to die within a month of birth as infants of normal weight
    (2) 7% of all births in 1977 were low birth weight
        (a) one in eight black babies were low birth weight
        (b) one in 17 white babies were low birth weight
    (3) low birth weight in newborns is related to inadequate prenatal care and a low standard of living
    (4) in 1978 almost 40% of black mothers received no prenatal care during the first trimester compared to 20% of white women

  b) health care provided for nonwhite and rural families is often inferior in quantity and quality to health care available to white and urban families
    (1) insufficient numbers of qualified health care personnel practicing in rural and poverty areas
    (2) inferior facilities for provision of health care are usually located in rural and poverty areas
    (3) a large percentage of health care offered to those living in poverty is provided by large institutions which tend to depersonalize the individual. This kind of care has discouraged early and regular attendance at prenatal clinics

  c) in many rural and nonwhite poverty areas, a low standard of living prevails
    (1) poor housing, sanitation, nutrition, and increased stress predispose mothers and infants to a higher incidence of morbidity and mortality

        (2) there is an increased incidence of pregnancies in adolescent mothers, leading to increased numbers of complications for mothers and infants

        (3) there is an increased incidence of out-of-wedlock pregnancies with concomitant problems

    d) lack of knowledge about health in rural and poverty areas decreases motivation to seek out adequate preventive health care

    e) maternal situational or economic deterrents

        (1) insufficient funds for transportation to clinics

        (2) ineligible for welfare and medicaid

        (3) language difficulty

        (4) cultural traditions that do not include medical care*

    f) the significant decrease in maternal and infant mortality between the years 1968-1979 may be a reflection of

        (1) increased federal and private foundation funding for maternal and child health services

        (2) increased use of monitoring devices during labor and delivery

        (3) increased dissemination of education about maternal and child health to consumer groups

        (4) accelerated application of research findings to maternal and child health care

8. factors contributing to improved maternal/child health in the general population

    a) economic: improved standard of living has led to better nutrition, housing, and health care

    b) environmental: improved sanitation has led to a decreased incidence of communicable diseases

    c) advances in medical science

        (1) blood typing has helped to control the complications of hemorrhage and blood incompatibilities

        (2) expanded pharmacological knowledge has facilitated treatment and prevention of conditions affecting maternal and infant health

        (3) increased knowledge about the complications of pregnancy has improved pre- and postnatal regimes of care

        (4) improved methods of providing analgesia and anesthesia has allowed for more comfortable and safer deliveries

        (5) technological advances, such as x-ray and ultrasonic pelvimetry, and fetal monitoring devices have reduced maternal and infant complications, through early and improved diagnosis of infant distress and difficult labor

---

*   Council of Scientific Affairs, AMA, Medical Care for Indigent and Culturally Displaced Obstetrical Patients and Their Newborns. JAMA, March 20, 1981, Vol. 245, No. 11, 1159-1160.

    d) improved education of health personnel in maternal and child care
       (1) specialized training for physicians
       (2) increased utilization of nurse-midwives for normal pregnancies and deliveries
       (3) the advent of the clinical-nurse specialist in maternal and child health
    e) improvement of hospital standards
       (1) accreditation has helped to upgrade standards of building, maintenance, equipment, and hospital care
       (2) infection control has reduced hospital-acquired infectious diseases
       (3) upgrading of qualifications of health care personnel employed in hospitals
    f) regionalized perinatal networks have been promoted by
       (1) federal "Improved Pregnancy Outcome Program"
       (2) Robert Wood Johnson Foundation
    g) high-risk pregnancies are detected early and referred to a specialized care facility in their region
    h) governmental and voluntary programs
       (1) 1900: census bureau established which provided accurate statistics on population trends
       (2) 1906: mortality statistics became reportable which facilitated the development of control measures for maternal and infant morbidity and mortality
       (3) 1907:
          (a) antepartal care was established through the Association for Improving Living Conditions of the Poor by providing nursing care
          (b) New York City milk supply improved through the dispensing of pasteurized milk
       (4) 1909:
          (a) American Association for Study and Prevention of Infant Mortality was established to study and correct the high infant mortality rates
          (b) first White House Conference on the "Dependent Child" resulted in
             1. the establishment of the Children's Bureau (1912) which conducted research and provided education to promote the health and welfare of children
             2. the establishment of child labor laws
       (5) 1912: first child health station was started in New York City to deliver primary health care
       (6) first use of prophylaxis in neonatal ophthalmia by installation of silver nitrate
       (7) 1919: second White House Conference reorganized the Children's Bureau
       (8) Sheppard-Towner Act: appropriated monies to improve health, welfare, and hygiene of mothers and

children through the establishment of educational programs for health personnel and lay people
(9) 1923:
    (a) Margaret Sanger Research Bureau for planned
        parenthood and infertility research and assistance
        started
    (b) Frontier Nursing Service was established in Ken-
        tucky (utilized nurse-midwives)
(10) 1930: third White House Conference - devoted to all
aspects of maternity and child care
(11) 1940: fourth White House Conference - devoted to
helping children grow into productive citizens in a
democracy
(12) Social Security Act (1935): Title V and Emergency
Infant Care Act
    (a) administered by Children's Bureau
    (b) extended services to local areas through grants in
        aid
    (c) enabled states to perform the following services
        by providing funds for
        1. establishment and operation of maternity clin-
           ics
        2. operation of prenatal classes for parents
        3. hospital maternity care for the indigent
        4. premature care centers
        5. public health nursing care for maternity pa-
           tients
        6. establishment and operation of well baby clinics
(13) 1945: United Nations World Health Organization (WHO):
maternal child health given top priority in importance
along with tuberculosis and VD as significant world
health problems
    (a) UNICEF established: provided emergency food
        and medical supplies to mothers and children
        where necessary throughout the world
(14) 1946: Hill-Burton Act provided funds for hospitals
expansion and set standards for accreditation
(15) 1950: fifth White House Conference devoted to needs
of children and youth
(16) 1954: Manual of Standard for Hospital Care of Newborn Infants established: improved conditions in hospitals for prevention of infant morbidity and mortality
(17) 1960: sixth White House Conference - focused on
problems of achieving full potential for youth
(18) 1963: amendments to Social Security Act - "Maternal Child Health and Mental Retardation Amendments"
    (a) increased number of prenatal clinics
    (b) brought clinics to the neighborhoods where they
        were needed
    (c) established high-risk clinics for prenatal care

(d) paid for hospital care, birth, prenatal care and delivery for the needy

(e) paid for hospital care of premature or injured babies

(f) supported demonstration programs in comprehensive child health supervision for families that lacked motivation

(19) 1970: seventh White House Conference - focused on children and poverty

(20) 1972: nurse practitioners functioning in extended roles

(21) 1973: Child and Family Resource Program: provides or makes available prenatal and nutritional education

(a) data demonstrated effectiveness of Rhogam in preventing RH sensitivity in RH-negative mother

(22) 1975: National Advisory Council of Maternal, Infant and Fetal Nutrition established

(a) WIC program implemented: provides low income families with supplemental food and nutrition education

(b) Title XX: amendment to Social Security Act provides comprehensive services which include family planning services

(c) National Health Planning and Resources Act: provides for coordination of health care services and resources

(23) 1979: designated as the Year of the Child by the United Nations to enhance care and well-being of children

## II. CURRENT PROBLEMS

A. Health care fails to meet the consumer's needs because it is
1. fragmented
2. uncoordinated
3. expensive
4. poorly distributed geographically and economically
5. impersonal and institutionally oriented

B. High maternal and infant mortality rates in nonwhite and rural populations

C. Maternal morbidity and mortality continue to be a problem
1. major causes of maternal complications include
a) hypertensive disorders of pregnancy
b) hemorrhage
c) infection
d) heart disease
e) diabetes
f) amniotic fluid embolism

D. Infant mortality and morbidity remains a problem
   1. major causes of infant complications include
      a) prematurity
      b) congenital malformations
      c) infections
      d) respiratory complications and asphyxia
      e) blood incompatibilities
      f) sudden infant death syndrome
      g) birth injuries

E. Syndrome of poverty influences the maternal and infant morbidity and mortality rates because it is associated with
   1. lack of education
   2. despair
   3. poor nutrition
   4. high birth rate
   5. lack of motivation to meet health needs
   6. poor housing and sanitation

III. WHAT REMAINS TO BE DONE ?

A. Removal of socioeconomic factors as a barrier to adequate maternity and infant care
   1. the syndrome of poverty must be treated

B. New methodology to improve the delivery of maternal/infant health services is needed

C. Provision of increased education to consumers about important factors in the prevention of maternal/child disorders is needed

D. Better utilization of health care personnel through expanded and changing roles and functions such as nurse-midwives, nurse practitioners, and clinical nurse specialists is required

E. Increased numbers of health care workers must be placed in areas where shortages exist

F. Systematic planning for coordination and distribution of health facilities must be instituted

IV. CHANGING CONCEPTS IN MATERNITY CARE

A. Family-centered maternity care began in the 1960s
   1. from conception until postnatal period the unit of nursing care is considered to be the family
   2. the rationale for the utilization of family-centered maternity care rather than obstetrical care is the impact that the pregnancy has on the family and the impact that the family

has on the physical and psychological well being of the pregnant woman

3. preparation for parenting is an essential part of maternity care
   a) family living classes are conducted in many secondary schools
   b) fathers and mothers attend preparation for childbirth classes
   c) fathers are included in the labor and delivery process
   d) rooming-in on postpartum units facilitates the transition to parenthood for mother and father
   e) research indicates immediate contact with the newborn after delivery promotes parental-child bonding
4. increasing numbers of institutions allow visiting by children to the postpartum unit
5. recently a new center for childbirth has been established in New York City by The Maternity Center of New York. This center provides a homelike setting for childbirth and demonstrates a commitment to family-centered maternity care

B. There has been an increasing trend toward home delivery in the past 10-12 years
   1. the lack of adequate medical backup in case of an emergency is of concern to both consumers and providers
   2. guidelines for family-centered care in hospitals has been developed by a multidisciplinary group so that the benefits of home delivery can be provided without the risks

C. Regionalization: increased technology and the concern about cost, quality and accessibility of care to pregnant women have brought about a trend towards regionalization
   1. level I agencies: usually at the community level are designed to provide services for the low-risk mother and newborn
      a) must be able to deal with emergencies until mother or infant can be transferred
   2. level II agencies: designed to provide an intermediate level of complex services and manage the more common complications of childbearing and the infant
      a) they are usually located in larger, urban, suburban communities
      b) act as a resource to level I institutions
   3. level III agencies: are able to provide a full range of all maternal/fetal and neonatal illnesses and abnormalities
      a) provide consultation services, transport teams, education and research to develop new knowledge in reproductive biology and related aspects of behavioral science
      b) evaluate functioning of the regional system

D.  Changing nursing roles
1.  nurse-midwife
     a)  gives total family-centered maternity care to the family
         unit in normal maternity
         (1)  responsible for
              (a)  prenatal period supervision
              (b)  management of labor and delivery
              (c)  postnatal care
     b)  the role of the nurse-midwife has evolved because of the
         need for increased comprehensive maternity care and
         the shortage of physicians qualified to give this care
     c)  nurse-midwives receive special preparation
         (1)  postgraduate education leading to certification varies
              in length
         (2)  master's degree programs which include certifica-
              tion
     d)  nurse-midwives practice in association with obstetri-
         cians
         (1)  work in obstetricians' offices in private practice
         (2)  employed by maternity centers, hospitals and com-
              munity health agencies
2.  clinical nurse specialist in maternity nursing
     a)  prepared at the master's level
     b)  acts as a role model and resource person for other
         nursing and technical personnel
     c)  assists parents in coping with special problems arising
         during the maternity cycle
     d)  functions in a teaching and leadership role
3.  maternity nurses
     a)  there is an increasing emphasis on anticipatory guid-
         ance, counselling and teaching throughout the maternity
         cycle in addition to the provision of safe, humanitarian
         care for parents and newborns

E.  Team approach to maternity nursing
1.  many levels of personnel cooperate to deliver maternity
     care to families.  Members of the team include profes-
     sional and technical nurses, nurses' aides, baby nurses,
     licensed practical nurses, physicians, and physician's as-
     sistants, nutritionists, social workers
2.  members of the team deliver the care for which their edu-
     cational preparation has prepared them

F.  There is an increasing dialogue between consumers and health
    care providers regarding the type and quality of maternity ser-
    vices being offered to the public
1.  consumers are increasingly demanding a real voice in the
     making of decisions regarding their care
2.  increasing dissatisfaction with the existing quality of care
     and the powerlessness of the consumer to effect change,

has led to an increase in the number of home deliveries,
self-care and health care by nonprofessionals

## STUDY QUESTIONS

1. Differentiate between the neonatal and perinatal death rates.
2. What factors contributed to the general reduction in maternal
   and infant death rates in the past 50 years?
3. Discuss briefly the contribution to maternal child health of each
   of the following:
   a. first White House Conference
   b. 1960 White House Conference
   c. Margaret Sanger
   d. World Health Organization
4. What are the factors that contribute to the disparity between
   white and nonwhite maternal and infant mortality rates?
5. What impact did the 1963 amendments to the Social Security Act
   have on maternal and infant care?
6. What are the leading causes of maternal mortality?
7. What are the leading causes of infant mortality?

## BIBLIOGRAPHY

Anderson and Lesser: Maternity in the United States, Gains and
Gaps, American Journal of Nursing, July, 1966.

Aponte, A.: The Syndromes of Poverty, American Journal of Nursing, August, 1966.

Bean, Margaret: The Nurse-Midwife Today, American Journal of
Nursing, May, 1971.

Committee on Perinatal Health: Towards Improving the Outcome of
Pregnancy, March of Dimes Birth Defects Foundation, 1977.

Cohen, Wilbur: What Makes An Effective National Health Program,
American Journal of Nursing, October, 1972.

Davitz, Lois: Childbirth Nigerian Style, RN, March, 1972.

Department of Health and Human Services: Public Health Service.
Promoting Health/Preventing Disease. Washington, D.C., Printing Office, 1980.

Donney, Ethel: Imagination in Maternity Care, American Journal of
Nursing, January, 1960.

Harpine, Frances: Concepts in Maternal Child Health, American
Journal of Nursing, December, 1961.

Klaus, Marshall and Trause, Maryann: Maternal Attachment and Mothering Disorders, Johnson & Johnson, 1975.

Lyons, A. and Petrucelli, R.J.: Medicine: An Illustrated History. N.Y., Harry N. Abrams, Inc., 1978.

NAACOG Bulletin, January, 1981.

Obrig, Alice: A Nurse-Midwife in Practice, American Journal of Nursing, May, 1971.

Reeder, S.J., Mastroianni, L., and Martin, L.: Maternity Nursing, 14th Ed., Philadelphia, J.B. Lippincott, 1980.

Rich, Olive J.: Hospital Routines as Rites of Passage in Developing Maternal Identity, Nursing Clinics of North America 4:101-190, 1969.

Rubin, Riva: Maternity Care in Our Society, American Journal of Nursing, July, 1963.

Russell, B. and Lofstrom, L.: Health Clinic for the Alienated, American Journal of Nursing, January, 1971.

Sweeney, Bernadette: Family-centered Care in Public Health Nursing, Nursing Forum Vol. IX, No. 2, 1970. pp. 169-175.

Surgeon General's Report Health: United States, 1980 National Center for Health Statistic

United States Department of Health, Education and Welfare, Promoting the Health of Mothers and Children, United States Government Printing Office, Washington, D.C., 1972.

U.S. Department Health, Education and Welfare, Child Health in America, 1976.

Wedenbach, E.: Family Centered Maternity Care, G.P. Putnam's Sons, N.Y., 1967.

Wegman, Myron: Annual Summary of Vital Statistics, Pediatrics, December, 1979.

World Health Organization: Technical Report Survey No. 51, Geneva, Switzerland, 1952.

CHAPTER 3

THE REPRODUCTIVE SYSTEM

I.    MALE ANATOMY AND PHYSIOLOGY (Fig. 3.1)

MALE REPRODUCTIVE SYSTEM

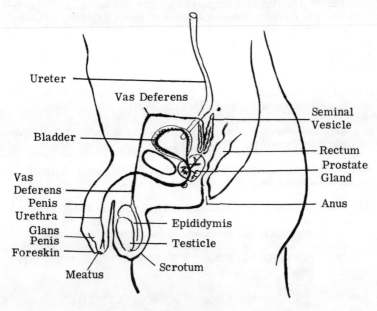

FIGURE 3.1

A.    Urethra
      1. passageway for semen from vas deferens through the penis
      2. passageway for urine from bladder through the penis
      3. the urethra ends at the urinary meatus which is the opening
         in the glans penis through which urine and semen are ex-
         creted

18

B. Testes
1. ovoid in shape
2. two in number
3. suspended in scrotum by spermatic cord
4. sperm formed and stored in seminiferous tubules of testes
5. testosterone is produced in testes

C. Epididymis
1. adjacent to testes in scrotum
2. acts as a storage reservoir for sperm in addition to semi-niferous tubules
   a) sperm may remain alive for as long as a month in both epididymis and tubules

D. Vas deferens
1. conducts sperm from epididymis to urethra

E. Seminal vesicles
1. secrete mucoid material into upper end of vas deferens
2. mucoid material helps to keep sperm alive and motile

F. Prostate gland
1. secretes alkaline fluid to activate sperm
   a) fluid is secreted into vas deferens
   b) fluid is milky and opaque and forms part of the seminal discharge

G. Penis
1. contains part of urethra
2. organ of copulation
3. divided into shaft and glans penis
   a) glans penis is most sensitive portion of penis
4. erectile tissue lies around urethra and causes erection
5. foreskin covers glans penis (removed by circumcision)

H. Bulbo-urethral glands (2)
1. secrete mucus during the sexual act
2. located on both sides of upper end of urethra

I. Sperm
1. testes produce billions of spermatozoa throughout the life cycle
2. sperm contains head, neck, body, and tail
   a) the principal components are
      (1) head which contains the genetic material of the male
      (2) tail which provides motility through flagellar move-ment (back and forth)
3. sperm move at a velocity of approximately 1 to 4 mm/min through female genital tract to seek the ovum
4. maturation of sperm cells (spermatogenesis)

        a) primary spermatocyte divided by meiosis to form secondary spermatocyte with haploid number of chromosomes (23)

        b) secondary spermatocyte matures into sperm cell

J.   Hormonal influences on male reproductive system
   1. hormones are essential to the mechanism of reproduction and to the development and maintenance of secondary sex characteristics
      a) testes dormant until puberty
        (1) anterior pituitary body secretes follicle stimulating hormone (FSH) and luteinizing hormone (LH) which cause growth and function of testes at puberty
      b) secondary sex characteristics are generated by increased testosterone production at puberty
        (1) growth of testes and penis
        (2) growth of facial and body hair
        (3) deepening of voice and widening of musculature of chest and shoulders

K.   Physiology of ejaculation
   1. sexual stimulation causes increased amounts of blood to enter erectile tissue of penis which thereby enlarges, causing an erection
   2. rhythmic peristalsis in genital ducts during orgasm causes semen to be propelled through epididymis, vas deferens, seminal ducts, and urethra
   3. semen
      a) consists of sperm and milky serous fluid from prostate and mucus from seminal vesicles
      b) 2.5-5 ml normal range secreted at each ejaculation
      c) each ml contains 20-150 million sperm
      d) total ejaculate may contain up to 1/2 billion sperm; minimum normal count is 125 million sperm per ejaculate
      e) contains fructose needed by sperm for nutrition
      f) prostate fluid highly alkaline, neutralizes acidic fluid from testes (sperm immobile in highly acid medium) and also neutralizes acidic vaginal mucosa

II.   FEMALE ANATOMY

A.   Pelvis (Figs. 3.2 and 3.3)
   1. contains generative organs, bladder, and rectum
   2. forms part of birth canal
   3. shaped like a funnel with a wide mouth
   4. divided into false and true pelvis by the inlet or brim
      a) sacral promontory and ileo-pectineal line are dividing points between true and false pelvis
   5. bones of pelvis
      a) consists of four bones joined together by
        (1) sacroiliac articulations

FEMALE PELVIS

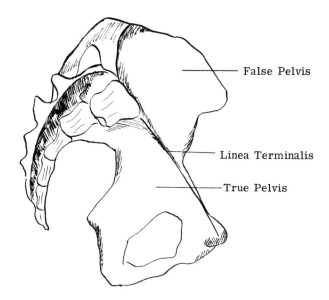

False Pelvis

Linea Terminalis

True Pelvis

FIGURE 3.2

    (2) symphysis pubis
    (3) sacrococcygeal articulations
  b) the bones of the pelvis are:
    (1) two innominate bones divided into three parts
      (a) ilium: flaring portion
      (b) ischium: lower part below hip joint
      (c) pubis: anterior portion
    (2) sacrum: posterior wall; pelvic portion of spinal column
    (3) coccyx: tail end of sacrum
6. inlet: heart-shaped entranceway into the true pelvis
  a) widest diameter side to side
  b) narrowest diameter: anterior to posterior
  c) measurements of anterior-posterior diameter are important in determining the course of labor
7. outlet: entranceway to vaginal canal for delivery
  a) irregular in shape
  b) contains soft tissue
  c) boundaries are sacrum, coccyx, symphysis pubis, tuberosities of ischia
  d) largest diameter is anterior-posterior, necessitating rotation of baby's head after leaving inlet in order for delivery to take place

## NORMAL FEMALE PELVIC MEASUREMENTS

INLET

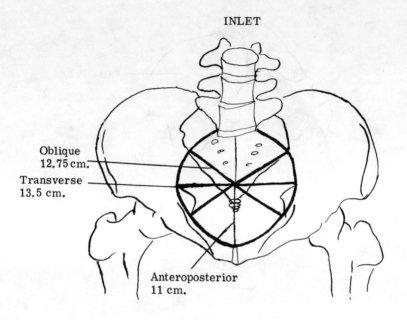

Oblique
12.75 cm.

Transverse
13.5 cm.

Anteroposterior
11 cm.

OUTLET

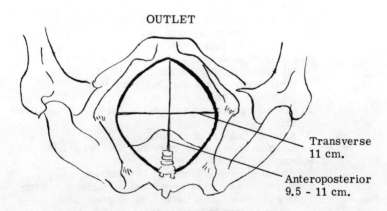

Transverse
11 cm.

Anteroposterior
9.5 - 11 cm.

FIGURE 3.3

8. soft structures of pelvis: ligaments, muscles, vagina, perineum
   a) form padding that protects the child
   b) form pelvic floor
      (1) retains pelvic organs in proper place

(2) directs presenting part of child forward during labor
9. pelvic types
    a) classification is determined by shape and measurements
    b) the type of pelvis will influence the course of labor and delivery
    c) classification system
       (1) gynecoid: anterior and posterior of pelvic inlet is well rounded; sacrosciatic notch is curved, moderate in width and depth
       (2) anthropoid: deep anterior and posterior inlet; sacrosciatic notch broad and shallow
       (3) android: wedge-shaped inlet, shallow posterior, pointed anterior; sacrosciatic notch narrow, deep, pointed
       (4) platypelloid: oval inlet, well rounded, with decreased anterior-posterior measurements; small sacrosciatic notch
    d) the closer the configuration of the pelvis is to the gynecoid shape, the more apt the labor and delivery will be normal

B.    Ovaries (Fig. 3.4)
    1. two glandular bodies shaped like almonds, on either side of the uterus
    2. attached by ligaments to pelvis
    3. contains primordial egg cells
       a) about 400,000 ova are present at birth
       b) contained in follicles
    4. surrounded by fatty tissue for protection

C.    Fallopian tubes (oviducts)
    1. attached to uterus on either side
    2. widens at ovarian end to form finger-like projections (fimbriae)
    3. acts as a passageway for sperm and egg (conception most often occurs in upper third)

D.    Uterus
    1. located behind bladder and in front of rectum
    2. nonpregnant state: hollow, pear-shaped organ weighing 50-60 g (2 oz)
    3. divided into three parts
       a) fundus: uppermost portion
       b) corpus: .body of uterus
       c) cervix: neck of uterus which opens into vaginal canal
          (1) internal os: opening from uterus to cervix
          (2) external os: opening from cervix to vaginal canal
    4. uterine wall made up of three layers
       a) external (exometrium)
          (1) continuation of pelvic peritoneum

## FEMALE REPRODUCTIVE SYSTEM

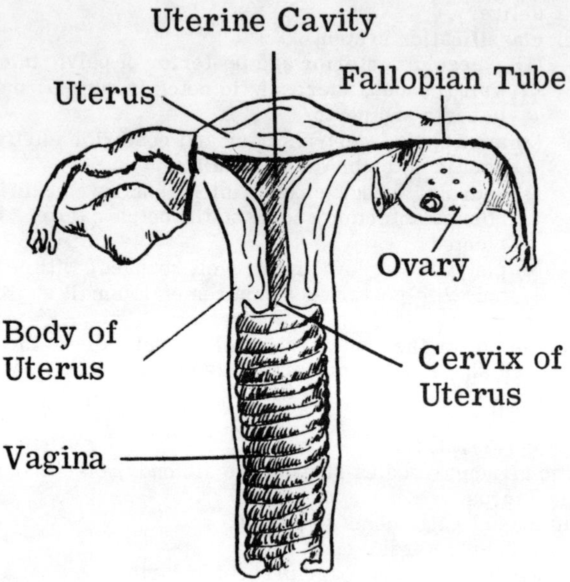

Uterine Cavity

Fallopian Tube

Uterus

Ovary

Body of
Uterus

Cervix of
Uterus

Vagina

FIGURE 3.4

    b) middle (myometrium)
       (1) contains a large number of blood vessels, nerves,
         and lymph vessels
       (2) extremely muscular
    c) inner (endometrium)
       (1) mucous membrane with rich supply of glands and blood
  5. suspended in pelvic cavity by broad ligaments

E.   Bartholin's glands
   1. two small glands on either side of vaginal opening
   2. secrete mucus

F.   External genitalia
   1. mons veneris: fatty cushion of connective tissue over sym-
      physis pubis
   2. labia
     a) majora: outer lips, protect inner vulva
     b) minora: inner lips, protect clitoris

3. clitoris: small projecting erectile organ
   a) well supplied with blood and nerves
   b) increases in size with sexual stimulation
   c) an organ of sexual excitement
4. vestibule
   a) space under clitoris and labia
   b) contains openings of:
      (1) vagina
      (2) urethra
      (3) glands of Skene's and Bartholin's
5. vagina: organ of copulation
   a) muscular, membranous orifice 3-5 inches long
   b) excretory organ of uterus
   c) birth canal
   d) hymen: fold of elastic tissue partially occluding vagina
      before first coitus
6. perineum: region from pubic arch to rectum
   a) forms external floor of pelvis
   b) provides muscular support for pelvic organs
7. breasts
   a) complex structures which function to secrete and con-
      vey milk to the nipples
   b) milk secretion takes place in lobes of breasts
   c) a system of ducts lead milk to nipples
   d) areola surrounds nipples and contains Montgomery's
      tubercles
   e) immediately after puberty, estrogen and progesterone
      begin to prepare breasts for lactation
      (1) breasts enlarge and glandular elements begin to de-
         velop

III. FEMALE PHYSIOLOGY

A. Hormonal cycle (Fig. 3.5)
   1. begins at puberty
   2. ends at menopause
   3. anterior pituitary secretes FSH (follicle stimulating hor-
      mone) which activates primary graafian follicle, allowing
      ova to mature
   4. increased estrogen is produced by maturing follicle
   5. estrogen stimulates endometrium to become engorged with
      blood and prepare to receive fertilized ovum
   6. estrogen and FSH allow ova to complete maturation
      a) primary oocyte forms secondary oocyte which becomes
         mature ovum with 23 chromosomes
   7. mature ovum is released through ruptured graafian follicle
   8. high estrogen levels reduce pituitary FSH and increase LH
      (luteinizing hormone) production which causes corpus lu-
      teum to secrete progesterone, which stimulates endometri-
      um to increase blood supply and store glycogen

## MENSTRUAL CYCLE

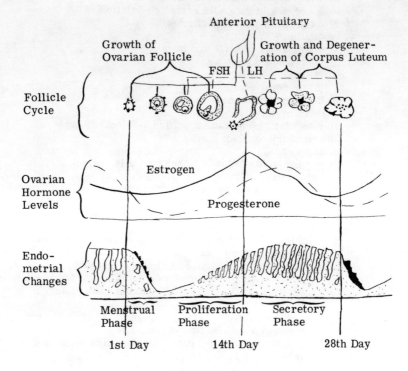

FIGURE 3.5

9. hormone levels drop and endometrium and corpus luteum degenerate
   a) progesterone levels increase and cause LH to decrease
   b) menstruation begins
10. usual range of menstrual cycle 21-35 days

B. Secondary sex characteristics develop in response to estrogen and progesterone secretion during puberty
   1. growth of axillary and pubic hair
   2. breast and genital enlargement
   3. widening of hips

CHAPTER 4

FAMILY PLANNING

I.  INFERTILITY

A.  Fertility rates
    1. highest in temperate zone
    2. 10 to 15% of married couples have fertility problems
    3. fertility diminishes with age
        a) peak of female fertility at age 24 with a gradual decline
           to age 30 and a more rapid decline thereafter to age 50
           (1) pregnancy after 50 is rare
        b) peak of male fertility at age 24 with a gradual decline
           (1) male fertility may remain as late as 80-90 years of
               age

B.  Causes of infertility
    1. genital tract abnormalities
        a) female
           (1) obstructions in genital tract from previous infection,
               injury, or congenital malformation of:
               (a) cervix
               (b) vagina
               (c) fallopian tube
               (d) uterus
           (2) tumors and cysts
               (a) vaginal
               (b) uterine
               (c) ovarian
           (3) allergic reaction to sperm cells
           (4) abnormal pH of vagina
           (5) endometriosis which is accumulation of endometrial
               cells either in the uterus or at other sites
           (6) endometritis: inflammation of the endometrium
           (7) infections or inflammation of any of the organs of re-
               production
        b) male
           (1) obstruction in genital tract from previous infection,
               injury, or congenital malformation of:
               (a) vas deferens
               (b) seminal ducts
               (c) prostate

          (d) urethra
- 1. hypospadias: urethral opening on underside of penis because of congenital malformation
- 2. epispadias: urethral opening on upperside of penis because of congenital malformation

    (2) testicle injury
       (a) sperm production may be affected by
- 1. radiation
- 2. undescended testicles
- 3. infection
  - a. orchitis: infection and inflammation of testes
  - b. venereal disease
  - c. mumps with a secondary infection of testes
- 4. trauma
- 5. hyperthermia: excessive heat applied to testicles
- 6. varicose vein in testicle

2. endocrine abnormalities
   a) female
     (1) pituitary dysfunction
     (2) ovarian dysfunction
     (3) thyroid dysfunction
     (4) luteal phase defect: when ovulation occurs after the fourteenth day of the cycle there may be structural changes in the ovum (sometimes labeled "over-ripeness") which may cause embryonic defects and abortion. Signs of luteal phase defects include delayed ovulation, shortened secretory phase, atypical temperature rise following ovulation, and other conditions
       (a) luteal phase defect may be a factor in infertility and habitual abortion
   b) male
     (1) testosterone dysfunction
     (2) pituitary dysfunction
     (3) thyroid dysfunction

3. systemic abnormalities in both male and female
   a) nutritional deficiency
   b) infection
   c) chronic disease
   d) fatigue
   e) emotional stress

4. sexual malfunctioning in male and female
   a) male impotence and premature ejaculation
   b) female vaginismus

5. chromosomal abnormality in male or female (Kleinfelter's or Turner's syndrome)

C.    Treatment
   1. genital tract abnormalities
     a) female

      (1) surgery
         (a) removal of obstruction, tumor, or cyst
         (b) correction of malformations
         (c) ovarian wedge resectioning for polycystic ovaries
      (2) tubal insufflation and hydrotubation for blocked fallopian tubes
      (3) desensitization methods for allergic reactions to sperm - condom used by male until antibody level of female drops
      (4) use of systemic and local drugs to alter abnormal acidic pH of vagina
      (5) treatment of local inflammation and infection
      (6) endometriosis may be treated by surgery or by suppression of menstruation through birth control pills for a period of time
    b) male
      (1) surgery
         (a) removal of obstruction, such as varicocele
         (b) correction of malformations
2. endocrine abnormalities
  a) female
      (1) current therapy for luteal phase defect which is in an experimental stage consists of inducing ovulation with a drug such as clomiphene and supporting the pregnancy with progesterone before implantation. This method needs further research because of the possible teratogenic effect of progesterone
      (2) methods used to determine ovulation occurrence
         (a) basal temperature chart is kept for several months
            1. temperature must be taken rectally for 5 min before getting out of bed, or doing some activity each morning (a specially calibrated thermometer is more accurate) a record is kept of daily readings. At the time of ovulation, there is a drop in temperature of from 0.5 to $1^{\circ}$ followed by a rise. There is a gradual return to preovulation temperature by the time menstruation occurs. Infections, severe stress or illness may affect temperature readings
              a. intercourse should take place at time of maximum temperature drop if pregnancy is desired
              b. if there is no definite pattern of a temperature drop and rise occurring during the cycle, ovulation may not be occurring
         (b) cervical mucus is examined for specific changes occurring during ovulation
         (c) an endometrial biopsy may be done to check for ovulation
         (d) Huhner test examines ability of sperm to swim in cervical mucus

        (3) drugs used to regulate ovulation
            (a) pergonal and clomiphene: to treat anovulation - stimulates pituitary to secrete FSH; may cause multiple pregnancies
            (b) birth control medication regulates menstrual cycle and may stimulate ovulation after drug is withdrawn
        (4) progesterone and estrogen have been used to correct deficiencies in hormonal production
            (a) the use of estrogen during pregnancy has been associated with the development of cancer of the genital organs in female offspring
            (b) it is suspected that sexual abnormalities in male offspring may be associated with estrogen use during pregnancy
            (c) the use of progesterone during pregnancy has been associated with the masculinization of the female fetus
        (5) poor cervical mucus may be treated with premarin or cryosurgery
    b) male
        (1) testosterone to correct deficiencies
        (2) pituitary, thyroid, or pergonal to correct deficiencies
        (3) if sperm count is low abstinence is advised for one week or longer to increase sperm count
            (a) first half of ejaculate contains the highest concentration of sperm
3. systemic disorders
    a) nutritional deficiencies corrected
    b) treatment of chronic diseases and infections
        (1) mycoplasmas (which are organisms somewhere between viruses and bacteria) are thought to be responsible for some cases of infertility
            (a) treatment with doxycycline has proved to be effective against the organism
    c) treatment of emotional stress
        (1) anxiety increases with prolonged childlessness
            (a) often spontaneous conception occurs after adoption
4. artificial insemination
    a) two types of artificial insemination are used
        (1) by husband
            (a) when sperm count is low or lacks sufficient motility, several ejaculations may be pooled to increase count
            (b) in order to bypass a highly acidic vagina
        (2) sperm obtained from donor other than husband when he is sterile
    b) procedure accomplished by injecting ejaculate with a syringe into mouth of cervix at time of ovulation
5. in vitro fertilization has been used to bypass occluded fallopian tubes

II.   FAMILY PLANNING

A.   Rationale for family planning
   1. overpopulation presents a threat to human survival
   2. individual desire to control size is influenced by economic, social, physical, psychological, and cultural factors
   3. adequate spacing of pregnancies decreases the incidence of maternal and infant complications

B.   The following methods have been utilized by individuals for family planning
   1. contraception
   2. permanent male and female sterilization
   3. abortion
      a) because of possible risk (6.1 deaths per 100,000 abortions in New York State in 1971 and possibility of cervix becoming incompetent after several abortions) it is advisable not to utilize abortion as a method of primary contraception

C.   Barriers to family planning
   1. lack of knowledge about effective methods
   2. misinformation about methods of family planning
   3. lack of adequate family planning facilities and personnel
   4. legal barriers to supplying services and equipment to minors
   5. lack of money needed to secure services
   6. religious and cultural attitudes towards family planning

D.   Family planning services available
   1. there has been a great increase in the funding and development of family planning facilities over the past 10 years by
      a) government agencies
      b) voluntary organizations, i.e., Planned Parenthood
   2. there has been a marked increase in research into more effective family planning methods. Funding for this research comes from government, private, and pharmaceutical companies' funds
   3. Medicaid has enabled many indigent people to obtain family planning services
   4. the Commission of Population Growth and the American Future was created by Congress in 1970 to develop a national policy on population growth
   5. in 1970, Congress passed the Family Planning Services and Population Research Act which authorizes funding for research and services in family planning throughout the country
   6. the Catholic Church has established clinics for research projects to instruct and improve the rhythm method of contraception

7. throughout the country, many public and private schools are introducing sex education programs into the curriculum which instruct teenagers in family planning
8. changes in state abortion laws and the decision by the Supreme Court that most state abortion laws are unconstitutional has resulted in a drop in the birth rate and a decrease in out-of-wedlock births

E.  What remains to be done?
1. safer and more effective methods of contraception must be developed
2. lack of knowledge and misinformation about family planning must be corrected by education in the schools and the community
3. family planning services must be made available to all, regardless of financial status
4. family planning services should be made available to minors who request them
5. quantity and quality of family planning services must be increased
6. maternal and child health nurses should develop the ability to counsel mothers about family planning on postpartum units, and prenatal clinics

F.  Methods of contraception: in choosing a method of contraception, a couple must consider effectiveness, compatibility and safety
1. coitus interruptus: oldest contraceptive procedure
   a) mode of action: male deposits semen outside of female genital tract by withdrawal of the penis prior to ejaculation
   b) acceptability
      (1) in the past widely used - currently it is decreasing in popular use throughout the world
      (2) requires no supplies or preparation, and no cost
      (3) makes great demands on self-control of the male, may interfere with sexual satisfaction of both partners
   c) effectiveness: varies with technique - with well-motivated couples who are adequately informed, it compares in effectiveness with other mechanical methods
      (1) semen must be deposited completely away from vulva as sperm may enter vagina from external labia
      (2) preejaculatory secretions may contain sperm in sufficient numbers to cause pregnancy
      (3) withdrawal must occur before ejaculation
   d) safety: no side effects have been proven, although many people believe mistakenly that this method can have physical or psychological effects
2. breast feeding: many societies have used prolonged lactation periods to space their families

a) mode of action: delays return of ovulation and menstruation
   (1) in order to prolong anovulation, major part of infant's diet must be breast milk
b) acceptability
   (1) not very acceptable in U.S. because of cultural attitudes toward breast feeding
   (2) used in many primitive tribes
c) effectiveness: prolongs anovulation for a certain period of time, but it is not always effective and ovulation may return before menstruation reoccurs, and pregnancy may result - not a reliable method
d) safety: no side effects

3. postcoital douche: widely used method in eighteenth and nineteenth centuries
   a) mode of action: plain water or vinegar douche used immediately after intercourse to mechanically remove semen from vagina. Vinegar used for spermicidal effect
   b) acceptability: inconvenient and ineffective; still used in U.S. to some degree by poor and misinformed
   c) effectiveness: least effective method used; sperm may reach cervical mucus 90 seconds after ejaculation
   d) safety: vinegar douche may change vaginal pH and secretions
   e) may speed the movement of sperm toward the cervix

4. vaginal diaphragm: widely used before advent of pill and I.U.D.
   a) mode of action: acts as mechanical barrier to the entry of sperm into cervical canal, blocking the cervical os. Used with a spermicide cream for additional protection
   b) acceptability: decreased popularity in U.S. since development of the pill and I.U.D.
      (1) must be fitted by a physician or health worker
      (2) must be inserted before intercourse. If intercourse does not occur within one hour additional spermicide should be inserted into vagina
      (3) many women dislike genital manipulation needed to insert
      (4) may interfere with spontaneity of the sex act
      (5) must be left in place after intercourse for six hours
   c) effectiveness: high level of protection - failure rate averages 2-3 pregnancies per 100 women per year if used correctly - if used without proper instruction, rate is much higher
      (1) reasons for failure are:
         (a) incorrect size
         (b) not inserted correctly
         (c) failure to use
         (d) tears or holes not detected in device
         (e) used without spermicide

    d) must be refitted after delivery, reproductive surgery and weight change that is significant. To maintain effectiveness size of diaphragm should be checked periodically

    e) safety: no side effects; rarely a woman may have a reaction to rubber or cream used

5. condom: used widely before development of pill and I.U.D.

    a) mode of action: covers penis during intercourse, and prevents deposit of semen in vagina; sheath is made of rubber

    b) acceptability: is presently used more frequently than the diaphragm in U.S., but has been replaced by pill and I.U.D. in popularity; protects against venereal disease as well as pregnancy

        (1) foreplay of sexual act must be interrupted to put on condom

        (2) may interfere with sexual sensations

        (3) may be purchased cheaply without prescription

    c) effectiveness: highly effective when used with spermicides; failure rate averages 3 per 100 women per year

        (1) FDA supervises standards of production and quality of condoms

        (2) high standard of quality exists in U.S. in productions

        (3) failures due to tearing or slipping off

6. spermicides: infrequently used as a sole method of contraception in U.S. Usually utilized in conjunction with diaphragm or condom

    a) mode of action: jellies, creams, foams, suppositories, and tablets containing spermicides are inserted into vagina before intercourse where they diffuse over vagina and cervix and immobilize sperm on contact. The spermicides also act as a mechanical barrier through which sperm cannot swim

    b) acceptability: not widely used

        (1) simple to use, do not need examination or prescription

        (2) vaginal leakage may occur (messiness)

        (3) several minutes of waiting must occur for suppositories and tablets to melt

        (4) creams, foams and jellies must be inserted with a tube applicator or sponge shortly before the sex act

        (5) effectiveness last on an average of one hour

    c) effectiveness: low rate of effectiveness; failure average 30 pregnancies per 100 women

        (1) quality of spermicides vary: foam is considered most effective form

        (2) amount inserted may not be adequate

        (3) uneven distribution of spermicide throughout the vagina

    d) no side effects; a woman rarely reacts to the chemicals used

7. rhythm method: includes calendar rhythm and basal temperature rhythm; only method of contraception advocated by the Catholic Church
   a) mode of action: abstinence practiced for a period of time before, during, and after the estimated day of ovulation
      (1) in order to practice the rhythm method, the day of ovulation must be determined
      (2) day of ovulation may be determined by calendar method or basal body temperature chart
         (a) calendar method depends on theory that the average ovulation occurs 14 days before first day of menstrual cycle
         (b) life of ovum is believed to be 12-24 hours after release from follicle
         (c) survival time for sperm is approximately 48 hours
         (d) considering all contingencies such as a variation of ovulation, the life of sperm and of ovum, the unsafe period is considered to be 8 days
         (e) a log is kept for a period of time to determine the longest and shortest length of a woman's menstrual cycle
            1. the shortest cycle is used for calculation
            2. 18 days are subtracted from last days of shortest cycle (14 days ovulation and 2 days variation in ovulation and 2 days life of sperm) this is first day of unsafe period; in a 28-day cycle, day 10 would be first day of abstinence
            3. to determine last day of unsafe period, 11 days are subtracted from last day of longest cycle (14 days ovulation and 1 day life of ovum); in a 32-day cycle, day 21 would be last unsafe day
         (f) basal temperature chart which is the more accurate method of the two is described under fertility. The time of abstinence would be 2 days before ovulation and 72 hours after the drop and sustained temperature rise. The reason for the 72-hour span is to be certain that ovulation has actually occurred. There are other small temperature fluctuations in the monthly cycle that are not related to ovulation. During ovulation the rise that follows the initial drop of 0.5 to 1° is sustained for at least 72 hours
      (3) methods of more accurately pinpointing ovulation are undergoing study at this time
         (a) fern test examines cervical mucus for fernlike patterns which occur prior to ovulation
         (b) spinnbarkeit test examines cervical mucus for evidence of thin and watery consistency and extreme stretchability which occurs prior to ovulation

      (c) Billings has developed a method of observation that can be utilized by women to determine when fertile mucus indicating ovulation is present

        1. during preovulatory period women are taught to check for appearance of increased mucoid secretion. At time of ovulation this secretion becomes clear, slippery and profuse. Abstinence should take place from the first appearance of cervical mucus until three days following the height of wetness

   b) acceptability: about one-third of practicing Catholics in this country use this method; a small percentage of women use this method for reasons other than religious

     (1) calls for a great deal of motivation, activity, and self-control for both partners

   c) effectiveness: basal temperature chart can be highly effective if done correctly and conscientiously, calendar method very ineffective; failures are due to

     (1) irregularity of menstrual cycle

     (2) lack of correct instruction about method

     (3) infections and drugs affect temperature readings

     (4) couples may not always practice abstinence when indicated

     (5) a small minority of women do not show significant temperature changes even though they are ovulating

   d) safety: no physical side effects; may cause anxiety

8. I.U.D. - intrauterine devices: widely used in U.S., Europe, and developing countries

   a) mode of action: a foreign body is placed permanently in the uterus where it exerts a contraceptive effect

     (1) exact method of action is unknown

     (2) theories as to mode of action are as follows:

       (a) causes speedup of egg's movements through fallopian tube, causing egg to reach endometrium before it had been completely prepared to accept it, and thereby preventing implantation

       (b) endometrial tissues react to the foreign body by creating toxic substances that interfere with implantation

       (c) stimulates cellular exudates that affect sperm mobility

       (d) may prevent implantation because of a nonspecific inflammatory reaction within the uterine cavity

   b) types of I.U.D.

     (1) early accepted devices

       (a) Dalkon shield - removed from market in 1975

       (b) Lippes-Loop-polyethylene - double shape

       (c) Safe-t-coil - double-coil plastic

       (d) older models were designed to fit entire uterine cavity

      (e) newer models of Lippes-Loop and Safe-t-coil come in various sizes to conform to uterine condition

  (2) modern devices
      (a) constructed of polyethylene (inert plastic)
      (b) smaller in size than older devices
      (c) can be used by women who have not borne children

  (3) types of newer devices
      (a) Progestasert: T-shaped, hollow device which gradually releases progesterone for a period of 1 year. Exerts a localized effect; no increase in hormone level of the blood has been found
      (b) copper 7 (shaped like a 7) and Tatum T (T-shaped) release small amounts of copper into the uterine cavity. Exert a localized effect; no increase in blood copper level has been found. Must be replaced in 3 years

  (4) women with the following conditions should not use an I.U.D.
      (a) fibroid tumors
      (b) pregnancy
      (c) pelvic inflammatory disease or a history of infection
      (d) abnormal pap smears
      (e) cervical disease
      (f) previous ectopic pregnancy
      (g) anemia or leukemia
      (h) allergies to copper
      (i) vaginal bleeding

  (5) I.U.D. may be inserted by placing it in a straight thin tube called an inserter. The I.U.D. is passed through the cervical os into the uterine cavity where the plastic resumes its original shape once inserter is removed. A thin thread remains in the vagina which enables the woman to check the placement of the I.U.D.

c) acceptability: would be an ideal contraceptive except for side effects and need for lower rate of failure. Widely used throughout the world
  (1) removed from sexual act
  (2) inexpensive
  (3) requires little motivation or education on part of user
  (4) extensively used in national programs in countries with population problems and low financial resources

d) effectiveness: highly effective method. Less effective than the pill. More effective than other traditional methods. Failure rate 1.3-5 pregnancies per 100 women
  (1) failure is often due to expulsion of device
      (a) expulsion rate highest during first menstruation and first four months after insertion

        (b) expulsion rates are higher when device is inserted soon after a birth
        (c) expulsion rates are higher in nulliparous women
    (2) women should be taught to check for expulsion
        (a) checking vaginally for placement of string or beads
        (b) after menstruation expulsion rates increase
    (3) pregnancy can occur with I.U.D. in place
        (a) in order to decrease possibility of septic abortion device is often removed when pregnancy is diagnosed
    (4) newer devices have lower expulsion rates
  e) safety
    (1) side effects include
        (a) excessive menstrual bleeding and bleeding between periods
           1. newer devices decrease bleeding
        (b) uterine cramping
           1. newer devices decrease cramping
        (c) depletion of iron from bleeding
        (d) increased incidence of ectopic pregnancy
    (2) voluntary removal rate is 36-34.8 per 100 users during first year
    (3) dangers include
        (a) perforation of uterus
        (b) women with previous histories of pelvic inflammatory disease may have recurrent flareups after insertion of I.U.D.
  f) the following factors affect failure, expulsion and complication rates
    (1) size and type of device and inserter
    (2) timing of insertion
    (3) insertion technique
    (4) skill and experience of inserter
    (5) follow-up care
    (6) counselling and teaching of client
  g) recent legislation now allows I.U.D. devices to be regulated by the FDA
9. oral contraceptives: most effective and widely used contraceptives in developed countries
  a) mode of action: synthetic compounds similar to natural hormones occurring in the menstrual and pregnancy cycle are used in dosages that prevent ovulation
    (1) estrogen blood level is low following menstruation. In a normal cycle low estrogen levels stimulate the pituitary gland to secrete FSH which causes an ovarian follicle to mature. The estrogen in the pill keeps the blood level high, preventing the pituitary from secreting FSH, and thereby preventing ovulation
        (a) progestin added to pills helps establish a menstrual cycle

(2) when pills are discontinued, withdrawal bleeding or menstruation occurs

(3) progestogen only pills are known to alter cervical mucous, interfere with implantation, and in some women suppress ovulation

b) types of oral contraceptive pills

   (1) combined pills: estrogen and progestogen are combined and are taken every day for 20 or 21 days of each menstrual cycle, starting on day five of menstruation

   (2) progestogen only pill

   (3) there are many different forms of birth control pills on the market. Each one may have a different dosage of estrogen and progestogen and each one must be prescribed by the physician according to the hormone profile of the woman. When breakthrough bleeding occurs during the cycle, the pill or the dosage may have to be changed

      (a) high or low estrogen types of women should take progestogen combinant pills that have an androgen reaction in the body

      (b) high or low androgen types of females should take estrogen dominant pills that do not have an androgen reaction in the body

      (c) when breakthrough bleeding occurs in the cycle the pill or dosage may have to be changed

      (d) high estrogen pills include Enovid 2.5 mg, Enovid 5 mg, Ovulen, Ortho Novum 2 mg

      (e) low estrogen pills include Ovral, Provest, Ortho Novum 1 mg, Norinyl 1 + 50, Brevicon

      (f) high progestogen pills include Norlestrin 2.5 mg, Enovid 5 mg, and Provest

      (g) progestogen only pills include Nor-Q.D. + Micronor and megestrol acetate

      (h) some types of progestogen in pills may react as an androgen in the body

         1. pills with androgen reaction include Ortho Novum 2 mg, Norinyl 2 mg

         2. pills without an androgen reaction include Ovral, Provest

c) pills must be taken every day for 20-21 days in order to be effective

   (1) if pill is omitted patient is told to take two pills on following day but there is a risk of pregnancy

d) acceptability: highly popular in U.S., especially among younger women with better than average education. Women with limited education can also be taught to use them effectively. There has been a decrease in use in the past few years due to increased concerns about side-effects

   (1) not connected with sex act

      (2) expensive compared to other methods - Government
          funding in U.S. has allowed distribution to low in-
          come women

      (3) simple to use, but does require motivation to take
          regularly

      (4) women who take pill need to be under regular medi-
          cal supervision because of the possibility of side ef-
          fects

e) effectiveness: most effective of all methods - combined
   type failure 0.1 pregnancy per 100 women, failure usually due to omission of a pill. Failure rate for progestogen only pill: 2.2 pregnancies per 100 women. The
   pills with the highest dosage of estrogen have the highest rate of effectiveness

f) safety

      (1) side effects include
          (a) nausea and vomiting, abdominal pains
          (b) breast engorgement
          (c) chloasma (brownish discoloration of skin)
          (d) spotting and bleeding between menses
          (e) fatigue
          (f) fluid retention and weight gain
          (g) amenorrhea
          (h) skin rash
          (i) loss of hair
          (j) vaginal discharge
          (k) headache
          (l) visual disturbance
          (m) acne

      (2) in attempting to eliminate side effects, it is impor-
          tant to be sure the patient is taking the pills correctly
          after a meal at the same time each day. Other causes
          for symptoms must be ruled out. If symptoms per-
          sist, the pill type and dosage may need to be changed,
          e.g., from a high to a low estrogen pill for chloasma
          and breast engorgement and from low to high estro-
          gen pill for acne

      (3) dangers include
          (a) an increased incidence of thromboembolic disor-
             ders and other vascular problems such as myo-
             cardial infarction, stroke and pulmonary embo-
             lism has been shown to be associated with the use
             of the pill. Death rate has been calculated to be
             5 per 100,000 age 15-34 years and 33 per 100,000
             users ages 35-44. However, the death rate from
             pregnancy in women age 20-34 is about 23 per
             100,000 women and age 35-44 is about 57 per
             100,000 women, and the pill is almost 100% ef-
             fective in preventing pregnancy. The death rate
             is increased in women who smoke and take the
             pill.

(b) it has been determined that the lowest dose of estrogen in the pill, 0.05 mg, has the lowest occurrence of thromboembolic disease
(c) blood pressure elevation in 5% of women on oral contraceptive
(d) increased incidence of gallbladder disease
(e) increased incidence of urinary tract infections
(f) increased incidence of eczema and sun sensitivity
(g) increased incidence of coronary artery disease
(h) liver tumors
(4) beneficial effects
  (a) decrease in premenstrual tension
  (b) regular menstrual cycle
  (c) shorter and lighter menstrual periods which may reduce the incidence of iron deficiency anemia in women
  (d) decrease in menstrual cramping
(5) contraindications
  (a) breast cancer
  (b) severe varicosities
  (c) phlebitis or embolic disease
  (d) hepatitis within the past 2 years
  (e) liver damage
  (f) severe hypertension (uncontrolled)
(6) the following conditions may or may not be a contraindication and must be individually assessed
  (a) diseases of heart, lungs or kidneys
  (b) diabetes
  (c) lupus erythematosus
  (d) arthritis (on steroid therapy)
  (e) sickle cell anemia
  (f) hyperthyroidism or tumors of thyroid
  (g) severe eye problems

10. male and female sterilization: a permanent method of birth control
  a) mode of action: cutting, ligation, or removal of portion of fallopian tubes in female, and vas deferens in male (vasectomy)
    (1) operation not usually reversible but some attempts at microsurgery have been successful
    (2) vasectomy may be performed under local anesthesia in physician's office; usually simple, uncomplicated procedure
    (3) tubal ligation traditionally performed under general anesthesia, using an abdominal or vaginal incision. Newer method is laparoscopy which may be performed under local anesthesia by inserting a laparoscope into the abdomen and severing the fallopian tubes through the laparoscope. Only a tiny incision is necessary, and patient may return home that day
  b) acceptability: widely used in India and other overpopulated countries. Vasectomy gaining in popularity in U.S.

      (1) a problem that exists with this method is the rare chance of reversibility if the individual changes his or her mind

      (2) if successful, operation leaves person completely safe from pregnancy

  c) effectiveness: failure rate varies with method used and technique of surgeon. If operation is successful, there is complete protection. In vasectomy there is a waiting period of approximately 2 to 6 weeks of active sexual activity for all sperm to be eliminated from the ejaculation as confirmed by laboratory test. It is advisable that forms of contraception be used until a sperm-free specimen is obtained. In a small percentage of vasectomies, the cut ends of the vas may rejoin

  d) safety: as with any surgical procedure, there is a risk to life

      (1) male surgery safer than female, although risk to both sexes is very low

      (2) vasectomy: complications occur in 2-4% of cases, and include

         (a) infection

         (b) hematoma

         (c) granuloma

         (d) epididymitis

         (e) no deaths have been recorded from vasectomy in the U.S.

      (3) tubal ligation: complications occur in 1-2% of cases and include

         (a) injury to bowel or uterus

         (b) excessive bleeding

         (c) mortality rate approximately one in 15-20 thousand cases and may be due to

            1. anesthesia reaction

            2. massive hemorrhage

            3. unrecognized infection of abdominal organs

11. morning-after pill

  a) mode of action: large doses of estrogen 3-5 days after intercourse

  b) acceptability: used only as an emergency measure because of hazards of large estrogen doses

  c) almost completely effective in preventing pregnancy

G. Possible future methods of family planning

  1. female

    a) once a month antiovulant injection: estrogen/progestogen combination is placed in a long acting steroid base, which lasts for a month

    b) continuous low-dose progestin administration

      (1) may be administered orally, by a subdermal implant, long action injection, or insertion of vaginal ring

        (2) has contraceptive effect without affecting ovulation or menstruation

    c) once a month antiprogestational pill: taken at time of menstruation and interferes with luteal maintenance of decidua

    d) immunization with sperm antigens to develop antibodies to sperm

    e) improved methods to detect ovulation through detecting LH or progesterone in saliva, urine, or blood

  2. male

    a) subdermal implant to suppress sperm production: low level androgen is constantly released from silicone rubber capsule

    b) periodic injections of long-acting androgen

    c) oral tablets of synthetic sperm production inhibitor: acts directly on testes to prevent the maturation of sperm

    d) possible reversible vas deferens occlusion and ligation

  3. unisex

    a) trials are presently being conducted on the use of a "superagonist" for both men and woman

        (1) peptide hormones are variants of the brain hormone LHRH (luteinizing hormone-releasing hormone)

        (2) prevent ovulation in women

        (3) prevent sperm production in men

## III. NURSING PROCESS IN FAMILY PLANNING

A. The emphasis for nursing as part of the total family planning team is to assist the family in planning and securing the desired family constellation

  1. nursing care in infertility

    a) assessment

        (1) period of time in which pregnancy has been actually sought

        (2) pattern of sexual activity

        (3) effect of infertility problem on interpersonal relationship of couple

        (4) effect of infertility problem on emotional health of each member of the family

        (5) identify external pressures from family and friends relating to infertility

        (6) coping patterns of couple with internal and external pressures

        (7) knowledge of process of conception and infertility

        (8) history of previous efforts directed towards treatment of infertility

        (9) ability of couple to understand the problem and explanations and instructions relating to the treatment of infertility

      (10) couple level of motivation in following through on diagnostic procedures and treatments

          (11) additional data is gathered from physical and laboratory examinations which will reveal possible causes of infertility

     b) nursing diagnosis

          (1) problems identified may include such things as

               (a) ineffective patterns of sexual activity (i.e., abstinence at time of ovulation)

               (b) anatomical or physiological abnormalities

               (c) inadequate coping patterns for dealing with internal and external pressures related to infertility

               (d) inadequate understanding of prescribed treatments or instructions

     c) goal setting: both long and short term goals should be developed collaboratively with clients and other members of the health team

     d) nursing intervention may include

          (1) teaching and counselling

          (2) assisting couple with identifying and changing their interpersonal relationship patterns

               (a) referral to appropriate health personnel may be necessary if problem goes beyond the scope of the nurse's competency

          (3) explanation of treatment and diagnostic procedures

          (4) assisting couple in exploring the implication and consequences of infertility on present and future life (i.e., adoption, artificial insemination, etc.)

     e) evaluation

          (1) the nurse should evaluate nursing intervention and goal achievement on a continuous basis

2. nursing care in contraception counselling

     a) assessment

          (1) client's knowledge of anatomy, physiology or reproductive system

          (2) client's knowledge of contraceptive methods and possible consequences associated with use

          (3) client's attitudes towards each contraceptive method

          (4) economic considerations

          (5) client's ability to understand and carry out instructions

b) nursing diagnosis is directed towards identifying potential barriers to successful use of contraceptive methods
c) goal setting: the nurse and other members of the health
team assist the client in determining which method of
contraception is best suited for her needs
d) nursing intervention: is concerned with teaching and
counselling the client in order for her to carry out the
contraceptive method of her choice
e) evaluation: return visits will allow the nurse to evaluate
   (1) client's understanding of how to use the contraceptive
   method
   (2) exploration of undesirable side effects or problems
   (3) client satisfaction with contraceptive method

# CHAPTER 5

## CONCEPTION

I. FERTILIZATION

A. Viability of sperm and ovum
1. sperm remain alive for an average of 48 hours after ejaculation
2. ovum remains viable for a period of 12-24 hours after ovulation

B. Fertile period is usually from 2 days before ovulation until 24 hours after ovulation occurs. For conception to take place sexual intercourse during this period is necessary

C. Fertilization
1. may occur in abdominal cavity just before ovum enters fallopian tube
2. usual place of fertilization is in the upper portion of fallopian tube
3. enzyme secreted by sperm dissolves outer covering of ovum to allow penetration of sperm
4. after one sperm enters ovum, the membrane surrounding it becomes impermeable
5. two nuclei, each with 23 chromosomes unite
6. fertilized ovum now called a zygote

II. IMPLANTATION

A. Occurs approximately 7 days after fertilization
1. during the period of the journey of the fertilized ovum, the endometrium, under the influence of progesterone, prepares for implantation
   a) becomes more vascular
   b) stores nutrients
2. the fertilized ovum begins to undergo cleavage (rapid mitotic cell division) soon after fertilization
   a) zygote is now known as morula
3. morula takes an average of 3 days to travel through tube
4. enters the uterus where it floats freely in uterine cavity for an average of 4 days, when it begins implantation
   a) morula becomes the blastocyst when it reaches uterine cavity

B. Blastocyst usually implants on the upper posterior wall of uterus
   1. outer portion of blastocyst made up of cells called trophoblasts
   2. trophoblasts penetrate into the uterine wall, digesting cells during its burrowing
      a) digested cells used for nutrition of the blastocyst
      b) the trophoblastic stage of fetal nutrition lasts until about the twelfth week of pregnancy when placenta is fully formed and takes over

III. AFTER IMPLANTATION

A. Endometrium becomes known as the decidua
   1. becomes thick and vascular
   2. stores nutrients and vitamins
   3. divided into three parts
      a) decidua vera: lines main uterine cavity
      b) decidua capsularis: surrounds the ovum
      c) decidua basalis: lies under implantation site; forms maternal portion of placenta

# CHAPTER 6

## FETAL DEVELOPMENT

I.  FETAL PHYSIOLOGY

A.  Placental development
   1. chorionic villi (finger-like projections covered with membrane) derived from trophoblastic layer of ovum
      a) penetrate uterine wall
      b) tap maternal blood supply, but membrane covering villi prevents fetal and maternal blood from mixing
      c) nutrients and waste products exchange by diffusion
      d) chorionic gonadotropin is secreted by villi
         (1) keeps corpus luteum from degenerating
         (2) enlarges corpus luteum which secretes increased amounts of estrogen and progesterone until placenta is fully formed
         (3) excreted in urine of pregnant woman by eighth to tenth day after fertilization and is utilized in A-Z, and Friedman Pregnancy tests
         (4) after full formation of placenta, chorionic gonadotropin production decreases, and placental secretions of estrogen and progesterone increase
   2. by the fourth month, maternal decidua basalis and fetal chorionic villi have formed placenta

B.  Placental function
   1. connects fetus to uterine wall
   2. organ of nutrition, excretion, and respiration of fetus
   3. secretes the following hormones:
      a) progesterone
         (1) sixteenth week, large quantities produced
         (2) causes endometrium to store glycogen, fats, and amino acids
         (3) inhibits uterine muscle contractions
         (4) aids in enlargement of breasts
         (5) causes increased reabsorption of sodium by kidney tubules
            (a) increases extracellular fluid and blood volume of mother
      b) estrogen
         (1) enlarges breasts
         (2) causes hypertrophy of uterine musculature

48

(3) aids growth and development of fetus
(4) controls development of female sex characteristics
(5) if estrogen production fails, fetus dies
    4. acts as protective barrier
      a) prevents some drugs and harmful organisms from entering fetal circulation

C.   Respiratory function of fetus
    1. some amniotic fluid components found in lungs of fetus
    2. most respiratory functioning occurs through placental circulation

D.   Digestive function of fetus
    1. digestive enzymes found in second trimester
    2. amniotic fluid swallowed after twelfth week
    3. meconium in intestine during second half of pregnancy
    4. most digestive functions occur through placental circulation

E.   Biliary function of fetus
    1. liver stores iron and carbohydrates from fourth month on

F.   Renal function of fetus
    1. capable of functioning, but not utilized because of placental functioning

G.   Fetal circulation
    1. distinctive features
      a) ductus venosus bypasses liver
      b) foramen ovale from right atrium to left atrium bypasses right ventricle
      c) ductus arteriosus shunt from pulmonary artery to aorta bypasses lungs
      d) umbilical cord contains umbilical arteries and vein which connect placenta to fetus
      e) hypogastric arteries return blood to umbilical arteries
    2. circulation pattern
      a) from placental blood vessels through umbilical vein, passing through ductus venosus (small amount to liver for nourishment), into inferior vena cava, into right atrium through foramen ovale to left atrium, to left ventricle, through aorta to fetal circulation of head and upper extremities, to superior vena cava, to the right atrium (mixes with blood from inferior vena cava), some to the pulmonary artery to nourish lungs, most through ductus arteriosus to aorta, distributed to lower extremities, abdomen and pelvis of fetus, to hypogastric arteries, to umbilical arteries to the placenta
      b) exchange of gases and nutrients in the placenta is accomplished by the process of diffusion
        (1) when blood in maternal sinus has higher pressure of nutrients and oxygen than blood in chorionic villi,

the nutrients and oxygen pass through membrane to
fetal blood supply by diffusion
c) maternal blood and fetal blood remain separate and
never mix, as they are separated by a membrane covering chorionic villi

H.   Amnion and chorion
1. membranes which surround the amniotic cavity
a) cavity contains amniotic fluid
(1) 1500-2000 ml at end of 6 months
(2) decreases after seventh month to 700 ml or less
2. amniotic fluid
a) functions
(1) cushions fetus against injury
(2) provides temperature stability
(3) allows fetus to move easily

II.   ANATOMICAL DEVELOPMENT

A.   Period of ovum: from fertilization to implantation, 5-7 days
after conception
1. 30 hours after fertilization
a) two cell stage
b) floating free in fallopian tube
c) reaches uterine cavity at 12-16 cell stage at which time
it is called a morula
2. 4 to 4.5 days: blastocyst forms
a) composed of
(1) inner cell mass; embryo proper
(2) outer cell mass (trophoblast); becomes fetal part of
placenta
3. 5-7 days
a) implantation begins
b) inner cell layer divides into
(1) ectoderm (outer layer)
(a) basis for development of
1. central nervous system (CNS)
2. skin
3. hair
4. nails
5. sweat and sebaceous glands
(2) mesoderm (middle layer)
(a) basis for development of
1. muscles
2. bones
3. kidneys
4. circulatory and reproductive systems
(3) endoderm (inner layer)
(a) basis for development of
1. liver

      2. pancreas
      3. digestive and respiratory systems

B.    Period of the embryo: from implantation to the completion of organogenesis (organ development); 8 weeks gestation
    1. end of first lunar month
      a) 0.25 in. long
      b) bent over itself
      c) spine formed
      d) beginning formation of
        (1) eyes
        (2) ears
        (3) nose
        (4) heart
        (5) digestive tract
        (6) arm and leg buds

C.    Period of the fetus: from completion of organogenesis to birth
    1. end of second lunar month
      a) head prominent, recognizable human face
      b) external genitalia present, but difficult to distinguish sex
      c) 1 in. from head to buttocks
      d) weighs 1/30th of an ounce
    2. end of third lunar month
      a) 3 in. long; about 1 oz in weight
      b) sex can be determined
      c) bones begin to ossify
      d) baby teeth buds begin to form
      e) fingers and toes begin to form
      f) fetal movement, not felt by mother
    3. end of fourth lunar month
      a) 6.5 in. long; 4 oz in weight
      b) external genitals obvious
    4. end of fifth lunar month
      a) lanugo: fine downy hair over body surface
      b) 10 in. long, about 8 oz in weight
      c) quickening: mother can feel movement
      d) fetal heart heard
      e) will make effort to breathe outside of uterus
      f) lungs insufficient to sustain life
    5. end of sixth lunar month
      a) 12 in. long; 1.5 lbs in weight
      b) considered viable: doesn't usually survive if delivered
      c) resembles miniature baby
      d) skin wrinkled: no fat pads
      e) vernix caseosa: cheesy substance to protect skin
    6. end of seventh lunar month
      a) 15 in. long; 2.5 lbs in weight
      b) better chance of survival if delivered

    7. end of eighth lunar month
      a) 16.5 in. long; 4 lbs in weight
      b) good chance of survival if delivered
    8. end of ninth lunar month
      a) 19 in. long; 6 lbs in weight
      b) well padded with subcutaneous fat
      c) survival same as term
    9. middle of tenth month
      a) 20 in. long; 7 lbs in weight
      b) skin white or pink
      c) lanugo mostly gone
      d) covered with vernix
      e) nails firm

NOTE: Length of full term varies from 240 to 300 days, usually 9.5 lunar months or 38 weeks.

III. FACTORS AFFECTING FETAL DEVELOPMENT

A. Sex determination
    1. female ovum carries only X gene
    2. male sperm carries either X or Y gene
    3. after fertilization
      a) if sperm contributes an X to zygote, sex will be female, XX
      b) if sperm contributes a Y to zygote, sex will be male, XY

B. Abnormalities of fetal development
    1. a large percentage of abnormal fetuses are expelled by spontaneous abortion
    2. infants who survive and are born with congenital malformations constitute approximately 3 to 5% of all live births
    3. the developing fetus may be adversely affected by genetic factors, or environmental factors
    4. genetic factors
      a) 23 pairs of chromosomes exist in each cell
        (1) 22 pairs are called autosomes
        (2) one pair is called the sex chromosomes
      b) chromosomes contain the genes
      c) during meiotic or mitotic division, abnormalities may occur producing a chromosomal defect
        (1) chromosomal defects may occur because of too much or too little chromosomal material in an autosome or sex chromosome pair
        (2) translocation and cross over of chromosomes may occur
      d) autosomal defects include:
        (1) Down's syndrome (mongolism): infant has 47 chromosomes as there is an extra chromosome at number 21 chromosome; this is called trisomy

(a) trisomy 21 usually occurs in mothers over 35 and is not genetically transmitted

(2) Down's syndrome can also be caused by translocation of chromosomes

    (a) translocation Down's syndrome is usually transmitted by a non-symptomatic mother with a translocation, and subsequent pregnancies may be similarly affected

(3) trisomy 13-15 and trisomy 17-18 also have occurred, causing severe abnormalities, and infants usually do not survive after birth

(4) autosomal dominance

    (a) a dominant trait that causes disease is present in the heterozygous state (Dd)

        1. few congenital defects are transmitted through autosomal dominance

        2. conditions are usually milder than recessive traits

        3. there is usually a wide spectrum of variation in the disease manifestations

        4. condition may occur as a result of a mutation rather than as an inherited gene

        5. autosomal dominant inherited conditions include:

           a. cleft palate

           b. polydactylia

           c. cataracts

           d. myopia

(5) autosomal recessive conditions

    (a) the individual with a congenital disease caused by a recessive gene inheritance is homozygous for gene (dd) (Fig. 6.1)

        1. both parents must carry the recessive defective gene Dd+Dd

        2. 50% of the children will usually be Dd asymptomatic carriers

        3. 25% of children will usually be normal DD

        4. 25% of children will be exposed to risk of the disease because they have dd-two recessive genes

    (b) examples of diseases and defects caused by recessive autosomal inheritance are

        1. inborn errors of metabolism

           a. protein disorders where defective or absent enzymes prevent metabolism of protein resulting in eventual death or mental retardation if untreated

           b. some inborn errors of metabolism are dominantly inherited or sex linked but the majority are recessive autosomal defects

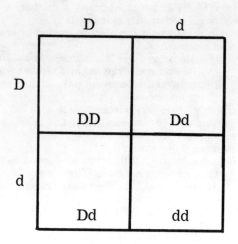

**DD - normal**
**Dd - carrier - no manifestations of disease**
**dd - disease**

FIGURE 6.1

   c. phenylketonuria (PKU) is a condition where
    the enzyme phenylalanine hydroxylase which
    is needed to convert the protein phenylala-
    nine is missing
   d. maple syrup urine disease (MSUD) and ga-
    lactosemia are two other examples of meta-
    bolic errors which have a much rarer inci-
    dence
  2. other autosomal recessive diseases include:
   a. diabetes
   b. Tay-Sachs disease
   c. muscular dystrophy
   d. Cooley's anemia
   e. albinism
 (6) sex chromosome abnormalities
  (a) one sex chromosome may be missing
   1. Turner's syndrome: one X missing, female
    appearance with few secondary sex character-
    istics
  (b) an extra X or Y may occur

        1. an extra Y or X chromosome does not necessarily result in abnormalities

        2. a male with XXY may develop Klinefelter's syndrome which causes sterility and testicular atrophy

        3. there has been some research which shows an association between XYY in males and aggressive or criminal behavior; subsequent research has not supported this

   (c) sex-linked defects

        1. recessive gene is carried only on X chromosome

        2. male does not carry corresponding dominant gene on Y chromosome to neutralize effect of recessive gene on X chromosome

        3. trait causes disease in males, but they cannot transmit it

        4. females are carriers but do not develop the disease

        5. example of sex-linked diseases:

           a. hemophilia

           b. color-blindness

5. environmental factors

   a) teratology is the study of the effect of environmental agents, e.g. drugs, radiation, pollution, and viruses, on the developing fetus, which may possibly lead to abnormalities

   b) principles of teratogenesis

     (1) the effects of the teratogenic agent depend primarily on the timing and intensity of dosage

       (a) excessive dosage of a teratogenic agent may kill the fetus

       (b) a dosage strong enough to affect the developing embryo and cause damage must be introduced into the mother at the time of maximum sensitivity on the developing organ in order to have an adverse effect

       (c) certain teratogenic agents may be neutralized by the action of other substances

       (d) the greatest vulnerability of a developing organ is at time of greatest mitotic activity during organogenesis

       (e) when organogenesis is completed, a teratogenic agent cannot cause malformation in the organ

       (f) the health and genetic structure of the mother may affect the activity of the agent

   c) types of teratogenic agents

     (1) components of normal body metabolism such as vitamins and hormones

     (2) chemical agents including drugs, gases, etc.

  (3) physical agents such as radiation, decompression, hypothermia, hyperthermia, amniotic sac puncture, and noise

 d) certain teratogens have been shown to be teratogenic in animals and have been strongly associated with fetal abnormalities in humans. Teratogens can also produce adverse effects on the neonate. Many additional substances are suspected of teratogenesis and continued research remains to be done in this area (Gullekson and Temple, 1978)

  (1) drugs

   (a) salicylates, and acetaminophen may effect kidney development and fetal bleeding

   (b) scopalomine: may cause early abortion

   (c) streptomycin: may cause deafness (eighth cranial nerve damage)

   (d) tetracyclines: may cause yellow teeth, slows bone growth

   (e) chloroquine: may cause deafness, damage to retina

   (f) anticonvulsants and barbiturates: may cause cleft lip and palate and other anomalies

   (g) thalidomide: may cause limb malformation (phocomelia)

   (h) meclizine: may cause cleft palate

   (i) anticancer agents: may cause cleft palate and other anomalies

   (j) amphetamines: may cause heart defects, cleft palate and other anomalies

   (k) caffeine, theophylline: may cause fetal tachycardia, liver damage, deficient clotting mechanisms

   (l) androgens, estrogens and DES: may cause masculinization of female infant or feminization of male infant, danger of cancer of vagina or cervix developing in women

   (m) corticosteroids: may cause cleft palate, club foot and other anomalies

   (n) magnesium antacids: may cause magnesium toxicity

   (o) sodium bicarbonate: may cause metabolic alkalosis, edema, fluid overload

   (p) psychoactive drugs: may cause bone anomalies, chromosomal damage

   (q) antidepressants: may cause a variety of anomalies

   (r) vitamin D: may cause a variety of anomalies including cardiopathies

   (s) narcotics: stillborn and drug addiction

   (t) alcohol

    1. fetal alcohol syndrome

     a. growth deficiency: small at birth, smaller

head circumference; remain shorter and
thinner as they grow older
   b. facial deformities: short eye slits, flattened
   nasal bridge, short nose and upper eyelid
   folds; there may be other anomalies
   c. CNS damage: slow development, lowered
   mental ability, may be hyperactive and ir-
   ritable
   d. not all babies of alcoholic mothers develop
   FAS (fetal alcohol syndrome)
   e. factors to be considered include duration of
   drinking and amount of alcohol consumed
   each day
   f. at the present time the exact relationship
   between amount of alcohol consumed and development of FAS has not been determined
2. smoking: may cause prematurity, low birth
   weights, abortion, higher rates of perinatal
   mortality, fetal abnormalities and placental
   abnormalities
3. "TORCH" complex of infections: toxoplasmosis, rubella, herpes simplex virus, cytomegalovirus, and other viruses are diseases that
   may be transmitted to the fetus and newborn
   which are capable of causing permanent damage
   a. toxoplasmosis: protazoal infection transmitted through the placenta which may cause
   growth retardation, immune deficiencies,
   hearing and eye defects and other anomalies
   b. rubella viral infection transmitted through
   the placenta can cause severe anomalies
   such as deafness, eye defects, and other
   anomalies
   c. cytomegalovirus (CMV): viral infection
   transmitted through placenta or through
   birth canal to neonate; may cause brain damage, liver disease, cerebral palsy and other
   anomalies
   d. herpes simplex (HSV): viral infection transmitted through placenta and through lesions
   in birth canal to newborn; may cause eye
   and CNS damage and other anomalies
   e. hepatitis B: viral infection transmitted
   through placenta and postnatally causes congenital hepatitis B in fetus and newborn
4. syphilis: bacterial infection can be transmitted through placenta or through lesions in
   birth canal; may cause congenital syphilis
5. x-rays: may cause congenital defects through
   radiation during organogenesis

6. heat: prolonged exposure to excessive heat may be harmful to the fetus; high maternal temperatures during illness or prolonged use of hot tubs may influence fetal development and prematurity
7. chemicals and gases: maternal exposure to lead, mercury, and anesthetic gases have been associated with fetal abnormalities

C. Nursing process to prevent fetal abnormalities. The emphasis for nursing is to observe for and to prevent abnormalities
1. assessment
   a) detailed family history to ascertain presence of inherited disorders
   b) history of possible teratogenic exposure of client
      (1) nutritional status and patterns
      (2) smoking
      (3) drug use
      (4) place of employment
      (5) exposure to radiation
      (6) infections and chronic illnesses
      (7) place of residence
2. nursing diagnosis is based on an evaluation of the assessment - possible problems identified include
   a) low protein intake
   b) excessive smoking
   c) familial history of an inherited disease
3. goals may include a
   a) cessation of smoking
   b) change in dietary patterns
   c) acceptance of possibility of a malformed child
4. intervention is directed toward limiting exposure to teratogenic agents, prevention of transmission of inherited diseases and assisting parents in coping with the possibility or actuality of malformations in offspring. Intervention may include
   a) advising caution about taking drugs during pregnancy unless it is absolutely necessary. Risk factors should be explored. Advise pregnant women to inform any physician who may prescribe drugs for a condition other than pregnancy, that they are pregnant
   b) recommending that x-ray tests be taken immediately after a menstrual cycle in women of child-bearing age and postponement of all other diagnostic x-ray tests that are not absolutely essential until completion of the pregnancy
   c) advising that women avoid exposure to infective diseases
   d) advising female children to be immunized against rubella before child-bearing age
   e) cautioning pregnant women against overdosages of vitamins and minerals
   f) advising discontinuance of smoking during pregnancy

g) instructing mothers how to maintain an optimal, physical and nutritional state

h) if it has been determined that exposure to teratogenic agents will actually result in an abnormal child - then intervention will include counselling to assist parents to cope with and accept the birth of the deformed child or termination of the pregnancy

i) if there is concern about the possibility of an inherited disease the parent should be advised to have genetic counselling

  (1) genetic counselling may include

    (a) karyotype (chromosome arrangement of single cell) of parents to determine probabilities of giving birth to an abnormal child

    (b) karyotyping of fetal cells obtained through amniocentesis may be performed. If abnormality is present, abortion may be recommended

    (c) enzyme levels of fetal cells obtained through amniocentesis may indicate presence of abnormalities

    (d) abnormalities that can be diagnosed in utero include Down's syndrome, Tay-Sachs disease, and maple syrup urine disease, among others

    (e) assisting parents in coping with feelings of guilt, helplessness and inadequacy that usually accompany genetic difficulties

    (f) assisting parents to make future plans and decisions such as adoption or childlessness

j) informing parents about the available screening tests for congenital defects

  (1) a blood test for pregnant women is now available which can detect increased alphafetoprotein (AFP) levels in the amniotic fluid. This protein passes through the placenta into the mother's blood stream. Small quantities of this protein are normal throughout the pregnancy. If a large quantity is detected in the blood test the possibility that the fetus has a neural tube defect such as spina bifida is considered. If a high level of AFP is detected a second blood test is is done, followed by a sonogram and an amniocentesis. If all of these tests point to a neural tube defect then the parents are faced with a decision of delivering a handicapped child or having a therapeutic abortion

    (a) it is extremely important that all three tests are done before making a diagnosis, as false positives may occur and other factors such as multiple births may cause high AFP levels

  (2) amniocentesis and fetal blood sampling may also be used to diagnose fetal defects such as

    (a) Cooley's anemia

 (b) Down's syndrome
 (c) galactosemia
 (d) hemophilia
 (e) sickle cell anemia
 (f) Tay-Sach's disease
(3) the increasing availability of prenatal testing brings with it many philosophical and ethical issues and questions relating to abortion
(4) there is a small risk to fetus and mother during amniocentesis
 (a) injury to fetus, placenta or cord
 (b) infection and abortion
 (c) risks are reduced when ultrasound scanning is used to pinpoint the location of fetus and placenta

CHAPTER 7

PREGNANCY

I.  PREPARATION FOR PARENTHOOD

A.  Healthy sexuality is related to the ability to relate fully to the
    opposite sex and the capacity to trust and love
    1. infant finds pleasure through sense of touch
       a) if pleasurable feelings are not distorted, a positive atti-
          tude toward sexuality should develop
       b) healthy sexuality develops from a childhood where de-
          velopmental tasks were completed and where basic hu-
          man needs were met
          (1) insures capacity of individuals to develop a trusting,
              open, caring relationship with others
    2. sex education
       a) correct information which imparts a healthy acceptance
          of human sexuality should be given as soon as child
          shows readiness
    3. parental relationships set tone for future sexual relation-
       ships of children
       a) a loving, caring relationship of mutual respect between
          parents encourages the development of healthy hetero-
          sexual relationships

B.  Attitude towards pregnancy depends on
    1. parents' childhood
    2. husband and wife relationship
    3. socioeconomic factors
    4. cultural factors
    5. knowledge about pregnancy
    6. fear of pain, hospitalization, etc.
    7. desire for parenthood

C.  Parental readiness for new role is related to their
    1. understanding of the parental role and a willingness to adapt
       to that role
    2. recognition of the uniqueness of children as individuals
    3. level of knowledge of basic stages of growth and develop-
       ment
    4. emotional maturity and family interpersonal and communi-
       cation skills

II. COMMUNITY RESOURCES TO ASSIST PREPARATION FOR PARENTHOOD

A. Maternity centers: provide counselling services, classes for expectant parents, prenatal and intrapartal services
1. nurse-midwives often provide care

B. Prenatal clinics: provide physical assessment and care during pregnancy. Psychological and emotional support is also provided

C. Classes for expectant parents are offered by
1. hospitals
2. community health agencies
3. maternity centers
4. Red Cross chapters
5. trained personnel from A.S.P.O.
6. course usually includes
   a) information about what to expect during pregnancy, labor and delivery, the postpartal period and the newborn
   b) encouragement of father involvement
   c) verbalization of thoughts and feelings of parents relating to parenting
   d) an attempt to reduce feelings of loneliness
   e) anticipatory guidance for parenthood
   f) preparation for labor and delivery
   g) preparation for new roles and new family developmental tasks

D. La Leche League is an organization of nursing mothers which encourages and assists others who wish to breast feed their children
1. chapters of La Leche League are organized in most major cities in the country
2. literature relating to successful breast feeding is available from the organization
3. regular meetings of mothers who are members of the organization are held in members' homes and are open to all
4. nursing mothers are encouraged to call fellow members of the organization whenever they need assistance or advice

E. Community Health Nurses: maintain prenatal clinics and visit families throughout the maternity cycle for counselling, instruction, and assistance in solving problems

F. Private physicians: assist in the maintenance of physical and emotional health during maternity cycle

G. A.S.P.O.: American Society for Prophylaxis in Obstetrics - classes given in Lamaze method of natural childbirth (for full explanation see page 150)

III.  PRENATAL REGIMEN

A.  Importance of early prenatal care
1. early diagnosis of pregnancy decreases possibility of complications
a) presumptive signs include cessation of menses, morning
sickness, tenderness and fullness of breasts, and frequent urination, Chadwick's sign, fatigue, fetal movement (quickening)
b) probable signs include enlarged abdomen, Hegar's sign,
ballottement, Goodell's sign, pregnancy tests based on
chorionic gonadotropin in blood and urine
c) positive signs: fetal heart beat and x-ray of fetal skele-
ton, sonagram, fetal movements felt by examiner
2. regular frequent maternity supervision allows early diagnosis and treatment of complications
a) decreases maternal and infant morbidity and mortality

B.  Prenatal health care delivery
1. the prospective parents are part of a health team that may
include one or more of the following personnel
a) nurse-midwife
b) physician
c) nurse
d) nutritionist
e) social worker
2. in many prenatal clinics the nurse functions as a coordina-
tor of the health team
3. each member of the health team delivers the health services that their education and experience prepares them to
do.  The nurse's role is carried out through utilization of
the nursing process

IV.  MATERNITY CARE DURING THE PRENATAL PERIOD RE-
LATING TO PHYSICAL NEEDS

A.  History and general physical assessment will help to determine if the pregnancy will proceed in an essentially normal
pattern or if the client or fetus is at risk
1. initial prenatal visit
a) physical exam
(1) history and general physical
(2) obstetrical exam determines general condition of reproductive organs
(a) pelvis evaluated for shape and size
(b) external measurements of pelvis determined
(c) vaginal exam
1. diagnostic tool to determine pregnancy
a. Goodell's sign - softening of cervix
b. Chadwick's sign - bluish hue of vaginal mucosa due to increased vascularity

    2. Pap test
    3. internal pelvic measurements
(3) breast exam
    (a) general condition
    (b) evaluation for lactation
(4) lab tests
    (a) urine
    (b) VD
    (c) blood
        1. cbc
        2. type
        3. RH
(5) calculation for estimated date of confinement (EDC)
    (a) date of first day of last menstrual period; add 9
        months and 7 days, or go back 3 months and add
        7 days (Naegel's rule)
    (b) length of pregnancy varies, making calculation
        difficult
        1. average length of pregnancy 266 days from
           time of conception
        2. average length of pregnancy 280 days from
           first day of last menstrual period (10 lunar
           months or 40 weeks)
        3. range of duration of pregnancy can be from
           240 to 300 days and still be considered within
           normal limit
(6) possible problems identified during the initial visit
    include
    (a) the presence of acute or chronic disease or dis-
        ability
        1. cardiovascular disease
        2. tuberculosis
        3. diabetes
        4. infectious disease
        5. venereal disease
        6. chronic debilitating disease
        7. urological disease
        8. anemia
    (b) blood incompatibilities
        1. RH factor
        2. ABO
    (c) pelvic abnormalities or disproportions
    (d) previous cesarians
    (e) history of previous difficulties during pregnancy
    (f) nutritional problems
    (g) history of previous premature births
    (h) adolescence
    (i) age over 35
    (j) high parity
    (k) socioeconomic status

(l) emotional problems of parents

(m) family interaction and role problems

(n) exposure to teratogenic agents

2. continued monitoring of physical status will allow for detection of any change in status of client and fetus. Examinations during return visits include

   a) abdominal palpation and auscultation to determine

      (1) size of fetus

      (2) position of fetus

      (3) fetal heart rate

   b) urine test to determine presence of

      (1) albumin

      (2) glucose

   c) weight determination

      (1) 25-28 pounds desirable weight gain for entire gestational period to prevent low birth weight infants

         (a) average weight gain during first trimester is 1.5 to 3 lbs monthly

         (b) average gain per week during second and third trimester 0.8 lbs

         (c) sudden sharp gain of weight after twentieth week of pregnancy may be danger signal of water retention and possible preeclampsia

         (d) approximate distribution of weight gain

            1. baby: 7.8 lbs

            2. placenta: 2.0 lbs

            3. amniotic fluid: 2.2 lbs

            4. enlarged uterus: 2.4 lbs

            5. enlarged breasts: 2.4 lbs

            6. increased blood volume: 2.4 lbs

            7. increased fluid in tissue: 5.8 lbs

            8. total: 25 lbs

   d) blood pressure reading

      (1) a sustained rise or fall of 15 mm is significant

   e) breast examination to assess condition of nipples and breast tissue

   f) vaginal examination in last trimester to determine

      (1) position

      (2) presentation

      (3) condition of cervix

3. significant symptoms that may be an indication of a problem developing include

   a) vaginal bleeding

   b) edema of face and fingers

   c) severe and continuous headache

   d) visual disturbances

   e) abdominal pain

   f) persistent vomiting

   g) chills and fever

   h) sudden escape of fluid from vagina

   i) a drop in hemoglobin or hematocrit

      j) presence of glucose or albumin
      k) abnormal or absent fetal heart sounds

4. nutritional assessment
   a) prepregnant weight patterns
   b) present weight
   c) color, skin turgor, signs of nutritional deficiencies
   d) presence of nausea and vomiting
   e) presence of any barriers to food ingestion (defective teeth, mouth infections)
   f) preexisting conditions that will affect dietary needs (e.g., diabetes, anemia)
   g) high risk factors relating to nutritional status
      (1) adolescents especially those with out-of-wedlock pregnancies
      (2) women with low prepregnancy weight and those who do not gain enough during pregnancy
      (3) women with a history of frequent pregnancy
      (4) women with low socioeconomic status
      (5) women who lack knowledge of good nutrition
      (6) women with a history of children of low birth weight
      (7) women with diseases which influence nutrition status (TB, diabetes, alcoholism, drug addiction, etc.)

5. sleep, rest, and exercise status assessment
   a) prepregnancy pattern of sleep, rest and exercise
   b) present pattern of sleep, rest and exercise
   c) complaints of fatigue
   d) opportunities for obtaining adequate sleep, rest and exercise
   e) barriers for obtaining adequate sleep, rest and exercise
   f) work conditions that mandate prolonged periods of sitting or standing

6. elimination patterns assessment
   a) prepregnant patterns of elimination - present patterns of elimination
   b) difficulties experienced with changing patterns of elimination

7. hygiene assessment
   a) prepregnant hygienic routines
   b) present hygienic routines
   c) presence of vaginal discharges

8. assessment of condition of breasts
   a) size, shape and discomfort
   b) condition of nipples
   c) plans for breast feeding
   d) are breasts properly supported

9. assessment of common conditions that may cause discomfort
   a) backache
   b) dyspnea
   c) varicosities

     d) leg cramps
     e) edema of lower extremities

B.   The rationale for nursing intervention to meet the physical needs of the pregnant woman is primarily based on the body changes that occur during pregnancy and needs of mother and child
   1. reproductive system changes
     a) uterus
       (1) increases in size from two ounces to approximately two pounds
       (2) changes from solid organ which has capacity of 2 cc to a thin-walled muscular sac capable of holding full-term fetus (approximately 7 lbs)
         (a) accomplished by hypertrophy of existing muscle cells and formation of new ones
         (b) estrogen stimulates hypertrophy of muscle fibers
       (3) increase in contractile ability
         (a) rhythmic contractions throughout pregnancy (painless and irregular Braxton-Hicks)
       (4) rises out of pelvic cavity
         (a) third or fourth month: palpated above symphysis pubis
         (b) sixth month: at umbilicus
         (c) ninth month: at xiphoid process
         (d) tenth month: in first pregnancy (primipara) uterus drops down (lightening)
       (5) as the uterus increases in size, the pressure on the abdominal wall causes the woman to walk with her shoulders thrown back and legs more apart to maintain body alignment
         (a) causes strain on muscles and ligaments of backs of thighs
         (b) muscular aches and cramps in late pregnancy
         (c) backache is caused by poor body alignment and relaxation of sacroiliac joints. Compensatory postural changes aggravate this condition
         (d) edema is common in lower extremities because of pressure of uterus on blood vessels
         (e) dyspnea is caused by pressure of growing uterus on diaphragm
         (f) varicose veins are caused by hereditary tendency and pressure in pelvis from enlarged uterus and on abdominal veins causing stasis of blood in leg veins. The stasis in leg veins causes thinning and stretching of wall of veins
         (g) frequent urination is caused by
            1. the growing uterus putting pressure on bladder until third month
            2. lightening, uterus again pushes against bladder

      b) cervix
        (1) softens in early pregnancy (Goodell's sign)
          (a) increased vascularization
          (b) proliferation of cervical glands which secrete mucus
            1. mucus plug expelled before labor
      c) vagina
        (1) increase in vascularity
          (a) gives purple hue (Chadwick's sign)
        (2) mucosa thickens
        (3) muscles hypertrophy
        (4) connective tissues loosen
        (5) increase in vaginal discharge
          (a) thick, white consistency
          (b) contains lactic acid; believed to help keep vagina free of pathogens
      d) perineum
        (1) increased vascularity
        (2) hypertrophy of skin and muscles
        (3) loosening of connective tissues
    2. breast changes
      a) enlargement
        (1) growth stimulated by estrogen and increased vascularity of tissue
        (2) progesterone changes tissue to secreting cells
        (3) growth of glandular (alveolar) tissue may cause pain and/or discomfort early in pregnancy
      b) nipples
        (1) deeply pigmented area surrounding nipple known as areola
        (2) erectile tissue
        (3) colostrum (precursor to milk)
          (a) thin watery yellow substance
          (b) appears after third month
      c) montogomery glands: embedded in areola sebaceous glands
        (1) enlarge during pregnancy
    3. gastrointestinal system changes
      a) distention of abdomen (mechanical)
        (1) striae gravidarum (reddish streaks) due to
          (a) rupture and atrophy of connective tissue of skin due to stretching
          (b) after pregnancy grow lighter and silvery white, like scar tissue
          (c) may or may not occur
      b) decreased peristalsis and muscle tone
        (1) hormones of pregnancy (progesterone) increase muscle relaxation and decrease gastric motility
          (a) constipation may occur if proper dietary habits are not practiced and if physical exercise is limited

c) hemorrhoids are varicosities of rectum and anus and may cause pain, discomfort and rectal bleeding
d) hormonal and metabolic changes may lead to nausea and vomiting (morning sickness)
    (1) symptoms usually appear between fourth and sixth week and may last until the fifteenth week
    (2) emotional factors are believed to influence the severity and frequency of the symptoms
e) heartburn is caused by reverse peristaltic waves causing backflow of stomach contents into esophagus
f) flatulence: usually caused by bacterial action in the intestine
4. hormonal and metabolic changes
  a) pituitary
    (1) anterior lobe secretes
      (a) lactogenic hormone after delivery
    (2) posterior lobe secretes
      (a) oxytocic hormone which allows contraction of uterus prior to onset of labor
  b) basal metabolism
    (1) decreases during first trimester
      (a) fatigue common complaint
    (2) increases during third trimester
5. nervous system changes
  a) altered because of hormonal changes
  b) variations in sensations may occur
    (1) neuralgias
    (2) pruritus
    (3) tingling
6. cardiovascular system
  a) blood volume – increased about 30% (Hydremia)
    (1) additional work load for heart – may lead to hypertrophy of heart muscle and poor circulation in extremities which can cause edema and varicosities
    (2) the highest level of cardiac output is reached during the 25th to 27th week
7. respiratory system
  a) last trimester dyspnea may occur
    (1) uterus pushes up diaphragm and chest cavity expands laterally
  b) vital capacity increased
8. urinary system
  a) kidneys – renal plasma flow increases approximately 20-25%, which increases the glomerular filtration rate 50%, causing increased urinary output
  b) ureters – may dilate because of pressure; more evident in right ureter
  c) bladder – increased pressure because of enlarging uterus (1st and 3rd trimester), causing frequency
  d) urinary changes may predispose to urinary infection

    9. skin
       a) striae gravidarum on abdomen, thighs and breasts
       b) linea nigra - brown or black line may form from mons
         to umbilicus
       c) chloasma (mask of pregnancy) brown blotches on face
         which disappear after delivery
       d) increased activity of sebaceous and sweat glands
   10. endocrine system
       a) chorionic villi
         (1) secretes chorionic gonadotropin until development of
           placenta (4th month)
         (2) maintains corpus luteum, to aid in proliferation of
           uterine lining, which in turn secretes estrogen and pro-
           gesterone (corpus luteum degenerates after 4th month)
       b) placenta secretes increased estrogen and progesterone
       c) pituitary body
         (1) anterior lobe secretes lactogenic hormone after de-
           livery
         (2) posterior lobe secretes oxytocic hormone which stim-
           ulates contraction of uterus prior to onset of labor
   11. muscular-skeletal system
       a) relaxation of ligaments and joints due to increase in re-
         laxin
       b) leg cramps are caused by decrease of calcium or increase
         in phosphorus. May occur at any time but are more
         common in late pregnancy
       c) body alignment changes may cause a posture imbalance
         leading to the possibility of the development of lordosis,
         backache, and varicosities

C.   Nursing care related to physical changes
    1. intervention is based on assessment data
       a) nursing care related to gastrointestinal change
         (1) assessment
           (a) degree of abdominal distention
           (b) elimination patterns
           (c) hemorrhoids
           (d) presence and degree of morning sickness
           (e) presence and degree of heartburn and flatulence
         (2) health teaching and counselling are directed towards
           alleviating present or potential problems
           (a) support garments may be required for pendulous
              abdomen
           (b) constipation
              1. increase of fluid intake if not contraindicated
              2. increase dietary fiber
              3. walking and mild exercise
           (c) hemorrhoids
              1. constipation aggravates condition and should be
                 avoided
              2. knee-chest position alleviates discomfort

        3. witch hazel compresses relieve discomfort
- (d) morning sickness
  1. use of small frequent meals during day and carbohydrate intake before getting out of bed in morning
  2. medication should be avoided if possible
  3. assessment and assistance in coping with emotional factors
- (e) heartburn
  1. restriction of fat
  2. use of alkaline preparations except sodium bicarbonate which promotes water retention
- (f) flatulence
  1. avoiding gas-forming foods such as beans, cabbage, etc.
  2. daily elimination

b) nursing care related to breast changes
- (1) assessment
  - (a) type of support worn
  - (b) usual care of breasts
  - (c) condition of nipple if mother plans to nurse
- (2) nursing intervention: health teaching and counselling
  - (a) good support is necessary due to increased size and weight of breasts
  - (b) cleansing of nipples without soap to prevent drying and caking of secretions
  - (c) massage of breast with cream may be indicated to preserve skin softness and turgor
  - (d) treatment of introverted nipples
    1. thumbs are placed firmly on areola close to nipple
    2. thumbs stroke areola toward and away from nipple horizontally and vertically
    3. repeated four or five times in succession

c) nursing care related to reproductive system changes
- (1) assessment
  - (a) posture and body mechanics
  - (b) edema of lower extremities
  - (c) dyspnea
  - (d) varicosities
  - (e) vaginal discharge
- (2) nursing intervention is directed toward client teaching and counselling for potential or present problems
  - (a) for muscle strain and backache
    1. good body mechanics, posture, rest, and proper shoes assist in relieving backache
    2. pelvic tilt exercises are helpful
       a. stand two feet away from support (back of chair or sink)
       b. bend forward at hip joints and place hands on edge of chair with arms straight

        c. raise hips and inhale

        d. round back, tuck buttocks under and exhale, knees should be slightly flexed

        e. repeat above three times

        f. drop hands and stand erect by raising breast bone straight up. Shoulders should be relaxed, knees flexed, buttocks tucked underneath, weight evenly balanced on back feet

    3. pelvic tilt exercises should be done twelve times a day

  (b) for edema

    1. rest and elevate feet to alleviate swelling

    2. prolonged sitting and standing aggravate condition

    3. careful evaluation is necessary since edema may be sign of hypertensive disease of pregnancy

  (c) for dyspnea

    1. sleeping in semi-Fowler's position will assist in relieving this symptom

    2. if heart disease is present, report any dyspnea to physician

  (d) for varicosities

    1. elastic stockings are used to prevent pooling of blood in leg veins and to provide support

    2. elevation of legs at frequent intervals assists return blood flow from extremities

    3. prolonged sitting or standing aggravates condition

    4. varicosities may occur in vulva and discomfort may be relieved by mother assuming an elevated Sims position (hips raised on pillow) several times daily

    5. anything that constricts circulation in legs should not be worn

  (e) for vaginal discharge

    1. douching prohibited

    2. personal hygiene important; perineal area should be cleansed from front to back

    3. discharge must be evaluated for possibility of presence of pathogens

d) nursing care related to urinary system change

  (1) assessment

    (a) any symptoms of infection

    (b) knowledge of self-care

  (2) teaching and counselling

    (a) adequate fluid intake is necessary to maintain bladder tone

    (b) immediate investigation of symptoms of infection

    (c) perineal area cleansing should be taught

e) nursing care related to skin change and general hygiene

(1) personal hygiene important to remove excess secretions
(2) explanation of normal skin changes during pregnancy
(3) regular dental hygiene should be maintained; dental
checkups. Bacterial growth in mouth may be increased
(a) dental x-rays should be avoided
f) nursing care related to changes in muscular skeletal
system
(1) assessment
(a) leg cramps
(b) postural imbalance
(2) teaching and counselling
(a) dietary adjustment or mineral supplement used
to alleviate leg cramping (calcium lactate or calcium gluconate)
(b) acute spasm can be relieved by forcing toes up-
ward and pressing down on knee
(c) exercise should be maintained to preserve muscle
tone
(d) good posture during pregnancy will prevent discomfort. To establish good posture the following
principles should be stressed
1. realignment of the pelvis tilting it toward posterior allows uterus to be carried more directly on pelvic bones
2. knees should be slightly flexed
3. pelvic tilt exercise assists in realignment of
pelvis
(e) heavy lifting and stretching become a hazard when
the body's natural alignment is altered
g) nursing care related to cardiovascular changes
(1) assessment
(a) BP
(b) fatigue
(c) edema
(2) teaching and counselling
(a) avoid fatigue when exercising
(b) take rest periods during day, avoid prolonged
standing or sitting
(c) elevate legs frequently
(d) avoid constricting garments
(3) sustained changes in BP must be immediately checked
by physician
h) nursing care related to nutritional needs of mother and
baby
(1) the quality and quantity of nutrients consumed by the
mother throughout her life will profoundly affect the
course of her pregnancy and the health of her child
(a) inadequate nutrition during childhood may interfere
with the optimal development of pelvic structures
in the mother

    (b) inadequate nutrition during childhood and adult-
hood may affect hormonal production and the menstrual cycle of the mother

    (c) inadequate nutrition during childhood and adult-
hood may affect the mother's health and well-
being

    (d) inadequate nutrition during childhood and adult-
hood may predispose the mother to maternal complications such as toxemia

    (e) inadequate nutrition has a direct influence on the
physical and mental growth and development of
the fetus

    (f) inadequate protein intake is associated with men-
tal retardation

    (g) inadequate vitamin and mineral intake has been
associated with bone and teeth deformities

    (h) inadequate nutritional intake has been associated
with increased incidence of low birth weight babies

(2) recommended nutritional changes during pregnancy

    (a) caloric intake should be increased approximately
300 K cal daily

        1. adequate energy is required for the develop-
ment and maintenance of new tissue related to
the pregnancy

        2. adequate energy is needed for the increased
activity level of the pregnant woman's increasingly heavier body as the pregnancy proceeds

        3. basal metabolic rates increase about 20% in
pregnancy

        4. adequate weight gain is needed to insure meet-
ing total energy requirements of the pregnant
woman and to insure an adequate birth weight
for the newborn

        5. obese women should not diet during pregnancy
but should maintain the required caloric intake
to assure fulfillment of energy requirements

        6. diet should be regulated to avoid excessive
weight gain

    (b) minerals

        1. calcium: increased by 0.4 g daily to a total
daily intake of approximately 1.2 g in the last
half of the pregnancy

          a. calcium is essential for the fetus

            (1.) to insure adequate development of bones
and teeth

            (2.) to maintain normal muscle action

            (3.) to maintain normal blood clotting mech-
anisms and myocardial function

        2. iron: requirements increase greatly during
pregnancy. Supplements of 30-60 mg daily
are recommended

       a. iron is needed for production of hemoglobin

       b. iron is stored by the fetus in the last tri-
mester to insure an adequate supply during
early infancy when inadequate iron is taken
in through the diet

  (c) protein: increased by 30 g daily to a total daily
intake of 76 g daily

    1. the rapid growth of the fetus, placenta, uter-
us, mammary glands and the increase in circulating blood volume account for the need for
additional supplies of protein

  (d) vitamins

    1. vitamin A: daily increase of 1000 IU is rec-
ommended to supply a daily intake of 6000 IU
in the last half of the pregnancy

      a. vitamin A is necessary for

        (1.) cell growth and development

        (2.) tooth formation

        (3.) normal bone growth

        (4.) integrity of epithelial cells

        (5.) overdosages of vitamin can produce
abnormal bone and liver changes

    2. B complex vitamins

      a. thiamine: daily increase of 0.1 mg to a
total daily intake of 1.1 mg

        (1.) utilized in the metabolism of carbohy-
drates

      b. riboflavin: increase of 0.3 mg to a total
daily intake of 1.8 mg

        (1.) essential for protein metabolism and
energy metabolism

      c. vitamin C: increase of 5-10 mg to a total
daily intake of 60 mg

        (1.) essential to develop connective and vas-
cular systems of fetus

        (2.) facilitates absorption of iron

      d. vitamin D: there is no recommended daily
allowance in adults for vitamin D. During
pregnancy 400 IU are recommended daily

        (1.) needed to facilitate calcium and phos-
phorous utilization

        (2.) overdosage of vitamin D intake should
be avoided as it has been known to
cause calcification of soft tissue primarily of lung and kidney

      e. niacin: increase of 2 mg

      f. vitamin B 6: increase of 5 mg

      g. vitamin B 12: increase of 1 mcg

(3) all other nutrients should remain at nonpregnant levels. Guidelines for choosing foods should be the basic four food groups

(4) in counselling women about nutrition during pregnancy the following factors must be considered
  (a) cultural background
  (b) economic status
  (c) individual dietary habits
  (d) presence of symptoms that affect food intake
  (e) educational level
  (f) motivation of mother for changing food habits
(5) to implement a change in dietary habits it is necessary to
  (a) obtain a diet history and daily log of food intake
  (b) motivate individual to assume responsibility for participating actively in plans for change
  (c) respect and accept all individual factors influencing diet habits
  (d) educate individuals about nutrition using terminology and techniques appropriate for their level of understanding

V.  NURSING CARE DURING THE PRENATAL PERIOD RELATING TO PSYCHOLOGICAL NEEDS

A.  Pregnancy usually occurs within the context of a family. The health and stability of the family will influence the course of the pregnancy and the pregnancy will have a profound effect on all members of the family

B.  Assessment
  1. readiness of parents for their new role; this readiness will depend on
    a) completion of developmental tasks of adolescence by both parents and assumption of the developmental tasks of the expectant family
    b) desire for parenthood by both parents
      (1) not all pregnancies are wanted
      (2) in some planned pregnancies there are fears and lack of confidence in ability to handle parent role
      (3) unrealistic conception of what it is to be a parent may impede readiness to accept a new role
      (4) cultural influences on concepts of parenthood and preparation for parenthood within the family group
  2. economic status of family may influence the family's acceptance of the pregnancy
    a) pregnancy may place a great financial burden on the family or may necessitate a change in the family's life style
      (1) living quarters may become overcrowded
      (2) working woman may have to give up her job
      (3) expense of having and supporting a baby may drain family's resources
  3. husband and wife's adjustment to marriage before pregnancy

    a) if either parent is unable to share the love and attention of the spouse, the pregnancy may become a threat to the stability of the marriage

    b) readiness of children in the family to accept a new baby

        (1) children who are insecure in their parents' love will be threatened by the arrival of a new baby

        (2) children between 18 months and 3 years of age may have particular difficulty in accepting a new baby since they are in the midst of resolving their own separation anxieties

        (3) children undergo a change in position and status within the family when a new baby is born

           (a) parental expectations of older children should not be radically altered because of the new baby's arrival

4. family relationships which are stress producing may affect the course of the pregnancy; pregnancy itself is a biological stress

    a) stress may be a causative factor in the development of

        (1) nausea and vomiting

        (2) hypertension

        (3) preeclampsia

        (4) postpartum psychosis

        (5) difficult labor

5. effect of pregnancy on the individual

    a) the mother's reaction to the pregnancy will be dependent on her individual

        (1) hormonal balance

        (2) state of physical health

        (3) emotional maturity

        (4) mental health

        (5) knowledge and understanding about pregnancy

    b) common emotional manifestations during pregnancy are

        (1) mood swings without relationship to external factors

        (2) increased irritability and sensitivity

        (3) changes in sexual drive (may increase or decrease)

        (4) introversion and passivity

        (5) narcissism (preoccupation with self and developing child as an extension of self)

        (6) disequilibrium between ego and id

           (a) ego control is diminished allowing id to surface

           (b) increased fantasy life

           (c) old unresolved problems surface

        (7) ambivalence includes acceptance and rejection of pregnancy

        (8) reaction to altered body image

    c) the father's emotional reaction to the pregnancy will be dependent upon

        (1) emotional maturity

        (2) mental health

        (3) economic situation

           (4) cultural preparation for parenthood
           (5) behavioral changes in wife that directly affect the husband-wife relationship
           (6) knowledge and understanding of pregnancy
6. communication patterns within the family
7. coping patterns of the family
    a) family strengths and weaknesses
    b) outside support systems
       (1) extended family
       (2) social relationships
       (3) community agencies
8. cultural background
    a) meaning of childbearing
    b) practices related to pregnancy
9. effect of pregnancy on sexual pattern and relationship
10. how realistic are the parents' expectations and goals regarding parenthood?

C. Intervention
  1. create an atmosphere in which the parents can verbalize freely about any possible or potential problem
    a) nonjudgmental attitude
    b) respect for cultural values
  2. allow sufficient time for the development of a therapeutic nurse-client relationship
  3. provide assistance to the client in identifying problems and setting goals
  4. the severity of the problems identified will determine the scope of intervention
    a) the nurse may provide information
    b) assistance in exploration of family communication and coping patterns
    c) provide support through empathetic and caring behaviors
    d) point out the strengths and support systems existing within the family and social circle
    e) provide sources and referrals for psychological counselling and therapy
    f) act as an advocate for the client
       (1) educate them as to their rights and privileges within the health care system
    g) act as a liaison between agencies

VI. NURSING CARE DURING THE PRENATAL PERIOD RELATING TO LEARNING NEEDS

A. Assessment of parents
  1. accuracy and completeness of information regarding parenting
  2. misconceptions about the maternity cycle
  3. level of ability to understand information and instructions
  4. level of motivation to learn

5. personal and cultural values which may influence acceptance of information and compliance with instructions

B. Intervention
   1. parents' classes may be recommended
   2. literature may be provided appropriate to the level of edu-
      cation and understanding of parents
   3. individual counselling and teaching by the nurse may be in-
      dicated
   4. teaching effectiveness is enhanced by
      a) choosing the time of optimum readiness for motivation
         to learn
         (1) information about labor and delivery process is
             meaningless in the first trimester of pregnancy
      b) limiting the amount of new information given at one time
      c) summarization and writing down important points
      d) providing feedback mechanism to assess learning
         (1) asking clients to repeat information in their own
             words
         (2) asking clients at frequent intervals if they under-
             stand material presented
             (a) verify by nonverbal cues
      e) provide an atmosphere where questions can be asked
         freely
   5. educational needs during the prenatal period may include
      a) anatomical and physiological changes of pregnancy
      b) labor and delivery process
      c) signs of labor
      d) nutrition
      e) signs of the development of possible or potential com-
         plications of pregnancy
      f) rationale for early and regular prenatal care
      g) safety precautions
      h) hospital admission and daily routine procedures
      i) hospital policies that affect mother-child-father inter-
         action
      j) rights of consumers of health care
      k) planning and purchasing of layette and other infant items
      l) preparation for natural childbirth
      m) prenatal exercises
      n) hygienic care
      o) fetal development
      p) general health care of self, e.g., rest, posture, cloth-
         ing, etc.
      q) care of the newborn

VII. NURSING PROCESS DURING THE ANTEPARTAL PERIOD
     INVOLVES THE ASSESSMENT OF PHYSIOLOGICAL, PSY-
     CHOSOCIAL AND LEARNING NEEDS IN TOTALITY, FOL-
     LOWED BY PROBLEM IDENTIFICATION, GOAL SETTING,
     INTERVENTION AND EVALUATION BY MUTUAL PARTICI-
     PATION OF THE CLIENT AND THE HEALTH TEAM

# CHAPTER 8

## HIGH RISK PREGNANCY

The term high risk is used to identify those women who may encounter problems or have preexisting conditions which may be detrimental to the outcome of the pregnancy. These women may need more intensive and frequent monitoring and care throughout pregnancy.

I.   FACTORS WHICH MAY LEAD TO A HIGH RISK PREGNANCY

A.   Socioeconomic status
     1. low-income parents face problems relating to
        a) adequate nutrition
        b) poor housing
        c) inadequate prenatal care
        d) sanitation
        e) untreated general health problems
        f) stress related to financial status
     2. implications for nursing process
        a) nurse may function as a consumer advocate advising about rights and making referrals where indicated
        b) nutrition counselling must reflect available resources
        c) nurse may facilitate utilization of prenatal facilities by recognizing possible and potential barriers caused by low-income status

B.   Age
     1. under 16
        a) nutritional status of adolescent girls may be below par, increasing the risk factor
        b) adolescents are in a state of growth and development themselves and pregnancy is an added physiological and psychological stressor that the body must adapt to
        c) higher incidence of hypertensive states of pregnancy and prematurity occurs in adolescents
        d) her schooling may be interrupted and she faces the risk of losing friends at a time when peer acceptance is most important
        e) implications for nursing process
           (1) assisting the adolescent in identifying and verbalizing her feelings about the pregnancy
           (2) assisting her to achieve the developmental tasks of adolescence

(3) helping her plan for postpregnancy life
(4) providing careful supervision and instruction about physical status during the maternity cycle to lessen danger of infant and maternal morbidity and mortality
(5) appropriate referral to social agencies whenever indicated

2. over 35 years of age
  a) higher incidence of complications including preeclampsia and fetal abnormalities
  b) increased rigidity of connective tissue
  c) hormonal levels may change
  d) childbearing at this age may cause emotional stress
  e) implications for nursing process
    (1) exploration of the meaning of the pregnancy to the family is important
    (2) careful monitoring of the pregnancy

C. Marital status
  1. out-of-wedlock pregnancy
    a) largest number of out-of-wedlock births occur in adolescents
    b) concealment of pregnancy may interfere with getting early prenatal care
    c) the adolescent father in an out-of-wedlock pregnancy often feels guilt and shame about the pregnancy
    d) the out-of-wedlock mother may have to cope with feelings of guilt and shame about her pregnancy and in addition may be rejected by her family
    e) changing attitudes towards premarital sex and out-of-wedlock pregnancy may significantly reduce feelings of guilt and shame
    f) implications for nursing care
      (1) woman should be assisted in making her decision about the placement of her child and support should be provided once her decision is made
      (2) if guilt feelings are present assistance may be needed in coping with them
      (3) the needs of the family of the pregnant woman and the father should be assessed and met

D. Parity
  1. five or more pregnancies
  2. implications for nursing process
    a) counselling about the possibility of precipate birth

E. Previous history of difficult labor

F. Reproductive system disorders

G. Accidents

H. Previous or current history of mental or emotional disorders
   1. preventative psychosocial support or therapy may be needed

I. Disordered family relationships
   1. family therapy may be needed

J. Previous or current history of complications during pregnancy
   1. hemorrhagic complications
      a) placental abnormalities
         (1) placenta previa
            (a) types
               1. total: cervical os completely covered by placenta
               2. partial: cervical os partially obliterated by placenta
               3. low or marginal implantation: placenta implanted at the opening of the os but does not cover it
            (b) etiology unknown but occurs more frequently in multiparous women who have had a rapid succession of pregnancies
            (c) symptoms
               1. painless bleeding usually in last trimester
               2. total placenta previa has earlier and more profuse bleeding
               3. premature rupture of membranes
               4. premature labor
               5. abnormal presentation
               6. delayed engagement
            (d) diagnosis is based on
               1. sonography (B-scan)
               2. radiographic (soft-tissue techniques, cystography techniques, ammiography, IV placentography
               3. manual examination of the internal cervix is rarely done because of danger of hemorrhage. If it is done, a "double set-up" is used
            (e) treatment
               1. hospitalization
               2. bedrest with sedation
               3. very restricted activity as blood clotting provides hemostasis
               4. treat shock, replace blood
               5. immediate delivery if bleeding is severe
                  a. deliver vaginally or by cesarean section, depending on placement of placenta
               6. constant observation
               7. if hemorrhage is controlled and pregnancy can

be maintained, cesarean section is usually
performed after the thirty-seventh week
(2) abruptio placentae
  (a) premature separation of the placenta before labor or delivery
  (b) etiology unknown: increased incidence occurs in
    1. hypertensive and preeclamptic patients
    2. violent labor
    3. uterine trauma
  (c) symptoms
    1. localized pain over uterus with or without hem-
orrhage
    2. uterus feels hard because of seepage of blood
between uterine muscle fibers
    3. maternal shock
    4. absence of fetal heart sounds
    5. couvelaire uterus may develop
      a. bluish, ecchymotic discoloration of uterus
caused by blood seepage into uterine walls
  (d) treatment
    1. hospitalization
    2. bedrest
    3. treat for shock and replace blood loss
    4. concealed hemorrhage may lead to afibrogene-
mia
    5. deliver vaginally or cesarean section depend-
ing on symptoms
    6. constant observation
    7. hysterectomy may be indicated in couvelaire
uterus
b) abortions
  (1) definition: expulsion of the products of conception
before fetus is able to survive
    (a) classification of products of conception
      1. abortus: 500 g and under
      2. immature: 500-1000 g
      3. premature: 1000-2500 g
  (2) types
    (a) threatened: cervix closed, may be stopped
    (b) inevitable: cervix open, certain to occur
    (c) incomplete: all or part of conceptus retained,
bleeding continues
    (d) complete: all of conceptus expelled, no further
treatment
    (e) missed: fetus dies in utero, but not expelled un-
til later months
    (f) habitual: three or more consecutive abortions
    (g) therapeutic
      1. medical indications (i.e., severe cardiac,
mental illness, TB, etc.)

2. on demand
   a. new statutes now permit abortion on demand
   b. Supreme Court decision in 1972 declared
      that statutes in states throughout the coun-
      try that prohibited abortion were unconsti-
      tutional. Women and their doctors may not
      be prohibited from making decisions about
      having an abortion
   c. reasons for women choosing to have an abor-
      tion
      (1.) unwanted pregnancy due to social, cul-
          tural, economic and psychological fac-
          tors
      (2.) may be used as a form of contraception
      (3.) to abort a suspected deformed fetus
   d. techniques
      (1.) early pregnancy to tenth week
          (a.) dilation and curettage is a dilation
              of cervix with a scraping out of
              uterine linings with a curette; gen-
              eral anesthesia is usually used
          (b.) dilation and evacuation (suction
              method): cervix is dilated and a
              suction tip is used to vacuum out
              contents of uterus; may be per-
              formed under general or local an-
              esthesia
      (2.) pregnancy after fourteenth week
          (a.) saline induction: hypertonic saline
              solution injected into amniotic sac
              through abdominal wall. Labor usu-
              ally follows 12 to 48 hours after in-
              jection. Patient must be hospital-
              ized. Performed under local an-
              esthesia
          (b.) hysterotomy: used after fifteenth
              week; surgical incision into uterus
              with removal of uterine contents.
              Usually accompanied by tubal liga-
              tion. Performed in hospital under
              general anesthesia
   e. dangers of abortion
      (1.) criminal abortions are abortions not
          performed by authorized health profes-
          sionals. These abortions may lead to
          hemorrhage, lacerations, perforation
          of uterus, infection and have a high
          morbidity and mortality rate
      (2.) complications for first trimester abor-
          tions
          (a.) perforation or cervical laceration

             (b.) bleeding
             (c.) complications of anesthesia
             (d.) incomplete evacuation
             (e.) infection
             (f.) RH isoimmunization in RH negative women
             (g.) cervical incompetence resulting in increased risk of spontaneous abortion and premature birth in subsequent pregnancies
          (3.) complications of 2nd trimester abortion include
             (a.) failure to abort
             (b.) birth of a live baby
             (c.) intravascular or intraperitoneal injection of hypertonic saline
             (d.) infection
             (e.) retained placenta
        f. nursing implications in abortions
          (1.) careful observation after procedure for complications
          (2.) pre- and postabortion counselling is essential to explore with the woman her feelings toward pregnancy and procedure in order to resolve any guilt or remorse over action taken
          (3.) a nurse who works in an abortion facility should be nonjudgemental
          (4.) Rh-negative women should receive rhogam after any type of abortion
  (3) etiology of causation of spontaneous abortion cannot always be determined
    (a) embryonic defect - primary cause
    (b) improper implantation
    (c) incompetent cervix
    (d) endocrine disturbances
    (e) abnormalities of the placenta
    (f) diseases and infections of mother
  (4) symptoms
    (a) bleeding
    (b) pain
  (5) treatment
    (a) bedrest
    (b) alcohol therapy
    (c) if bleeding continues, D&C is done
    (d) treat for hemorrhage and shock if necessary
    (e) treatment of habitual abortions
      1. determination of etiology is essential
        a. most common causes are
          (1.) incompetent cervix
          (2.) hormonal dysfunction

     (3.) abnormalities of uterus
     (4.) luteal phase defect
   2. luteal phase defect is treated by inducing ovulation with clomiphene and encouraging immediate fertilization. The pregnancy is then supported by progestin administration until implantation takes place (Grant, 1976)
   3. hormonal treatment especially with synthetic estrogens is strongly contraindicated because of highly increased incidences of vaginal carcinomas in female offspring
   4. treatment for incompetent cervix (inability of internal os to remain undilated)
    a. cervix is sutured to prevent dilation and removed 2 to 3 weeks before term
    b. bedrest
 c) ectopic or extrauterine pregnancy
  (1) tubal
   (a) occurs in 1 in 300 pregnancies
   (b) cause believed to be tubal malformations and defects arising from genetic or infectious origins and use of I.U.D. for contraception
   (c) prognosis: may rupture or abort or may be propelled out into abdominal cavity
   (d) symptoms
    1. unruptured
     a. menstrual abnormality, amenorrhea or spotting. Menses rarely remain normal
     b. lower abdominal pain midline or unilateral
     c. symptoms of pregnancy
    2. ruptured
     a. severe pain during rupture
     b. after rupture, referred pain to shoulder
     c. syncope, shock
     d. unable to void
     e. rectal pressure
     f. external bleeding not profuse
     g. occurs 5-6 weeks after last menstrual period
   (e) treatment
    1. treat hemorrhage and shock
    2. surgery
    3. sometimes tube can be repaired
  (2) abdominal pregnancy
   (a) rare: 1 in 15,000
   (b) may have symptoms of tubal or normal pregnancy
   (c) 20% carry to term; delivered by surgery
   (d) danger of hemorrhage and infection
   (e) on delivery, placenta left in place and absorbed
  (3) interstitial and ovarian pregnancies are extremely rare

d) gestational trophoblastic disease (Tiku, 1978)
  (1) molar pregnancy: hydatidiform mole may be
    (a) invasive
    (b) noninvasive
  (2) associated with pathological conceptus in which the embryo is absent or dead prior to time of establishment of fetal circulation
  (3) trophoblastic proliferation occurs with edema of connective tissue stroma
  (4) in invasive mole there is a large amount of trophoblastic overgrowth and a large amount of penetration of the villi into the uterine wall
  (5) danger of developing into choriocarcinoma which is an epithelial tumor of the embryonic chorion which is subject to early and widespread metastases
  (6) prognosis
    (a) 80% of hydatidiform moles have a benign course
    (b) 16% become invasive moles
    (c) 2.5% progress to choriocarcinoma
  (7) etiology: unknown
    (a) more common in Far East (1:700); rate in U.S. is 1:2000
    (b) more prevalent in women over 40
  (8) diagnosis
    (a) immunoassays to detect titer of
      1. human chorionic gonadotropin (HCG)
        a. in normal pregnancy peak excretion is 10-12 weeks, then it drops. In molar pregnancies, usually HCG fails to drop or rises markedly
      2. human placental lactogen (HPL)
        a. is usually lower in molar pregnancy
    (b) sonography (beta scan)
    (c) radiographic technique
  (9) symptoms
    (a) excessive nausea and vomiting
    (b) rapid enlargement of uterus
    (c) amenorrhea followed by intermittent bleeding usually accompanied by grapelike vesicles
    (d) absence of fetal heart tones
  (10) treatment
    (a) removal by D&C or vacuum aspiration
    (b) if excessive bleeding has occurred a blood transfusion may be needed
    (c) follow-up care
      1. pregnancy should be avoided for 1 year
      2. weekly tests for HCG titers
        a. negative titers should occur within 6 weeks after removal
        b. increased titers may indicate development of chorionic malignancy

           3. uterine bleeding, failure of uterus to contract or signs of metastatic tumors may indicate chorionic malignancy (chest x-rays should be taken at 4 and 8 weeks post-D&C)

      (d) choriocarcinoma can be treated successfully with chemotherapy

  e) nursing care in hemorrhagic complications

    (1) assessment includes

      (a) observation of vital signs

      (b) amount and character of bleeding

        1. amount

        2. color

        3. rate of flow

        4. clots or tissue passed (save for examination by physician)

      (c) emotional reaction to condition

      (d) reaction to prescribed treatment

    (2) intervention includes

      (a) prevention of infection

      (b) save expelled tissue

      (c) prevent shock

      (d) maintain fluid and electrolyte balance

      (e) provide support to patient throughout the experience

      (f) provide adequate and accurate information to patients

      (g) provide a climate for verbalization of feelings

2. hydramnios

  a) polyhydramnios: excessive quantity of amniotic fluid

    (1) normal volume 1000 cc, over 2000 cc considered excessive

    (2) etiology unknown, associated with

      (a) multiple births

      (b) fetal malformation

      (c) hydrops fetalis

      (d) preeclampsia

      (e) may be related to inability of the fetus to swallow amniotic fluid

    (3) symptoms due to the increased pressure exerted by the uterus on nearby organs

      (a) respiratory distress

      (b) edema of abdominal wall, vulva, and lower extremities

      (c) uterine pain

      (d) nausea and vomiting

    (4) diagnosis

      (a) excessive uterine enlargement

      (b) difficulty in hearing fetal heart tones, and palpation of fetus

      (c) ease of ballottement: testing for the rebound of fetus when pressure is applied to it through its

                fluid medium
    (d) increased fetal activity
    (e) sonography
    (f) radiography
  (5) management
    (a) amniocentesis: removal of amniotic fluid from uterus through insertion of needle through the abdomen into the amniotic sac
  b) oligohydramnios: small amount of amniotic fluid
    (1) volume less than 100 cc
    (2) in early pregnancy may cause amnion to come in contact with fetus and adhesion occurs
    (3) during labor first stage is prolonged because of decrease in hydrostatic pressure from amniotic fluid
  c) implications for nursing care in polyhydramnios
    (1) adequate information regarding the physiological basis for her symptoms
    (2) semi-Fowler position may relieve dyspnea
    (3) adequate abdominal support
    (4) adequate explanations of treatment regimen
3. hyperemesis gravidarum: pernicious vomiting
  a) etiology unknown but thought to be related to
    (1) hormonal changes; high levels of HCG
    (2) maladjustment of maternal metabolism
    (3) change in gastric motility
    (4) toxicity
    (5) psychic factors
  b) symptoms
    (1) pernicious vomiting
    (2) dehydration
    (3) marked weight loss
    (4) ketosis
    (5) rapid pulse (over 100)
    (6) hypertension
    (7) electrolyte imbalance
  c) treatment
    (1) adequate care of morning sickness may prevent condition
    (2) hospitalization
      (a) bedrest
      (b) sedation
      (c) IV or hyperalimentation therapy
        1. prevents dehydration and starvation
      (d) vitamin therapy (emphasis on B 6)
      (e) psychological counselling
      (f) careful observation of intake and output
  d) implications for nursing care
    (1) assessment of fluid and electrolyte needs
    (2) hygienic care after vomiting
    (3) provide opportunity for adequate rest
    (4) allow for verbalization of feelings regarding pregnancy

    4. blood incompatibilities
      a) Rh factor
        (1) etiology: when Rh-negative mother conceives baby
            with Rh-positive father
           (a) high incidence of Rh-positive babies because of
               dominance of Rh-positive factor gene
           (b) sensitization of mother to Rh factor with produc-
               tion of antibodies occurs during labor and deliv-
               ery of first baby or previous blood transfusions
               with Rh-positive blood
           (c) during subsequent pregnancies, antibodies of
               mother pass through placenta to fetus causing de-
               struction of fetal red blood cells
              1. condition may be mild to severe, and results
                  can range from anemia to hydrops fetalis in
                  utero, and kernicterus in the neonate
        (2) management
           (a) prevention of antibody development in mother by
               Rhogam, a vaccine that prevents sensitization
              1. must be given before 72 hours after delivery
                  or abortion
              2. vaccine ineffective after sensitization of moth-
                  er has occurred
           (b) if mother has been sensitized
              1. mother's antibody level is monitored
              2. if antibody level is increased, an intrauterine
                  blood transfusion of fetus may be done
           (c) management of neonate
              1. frequent monitoring of bilirubin levels
              2. if bilirubin level rises above normal, exchange
                  transfusion may be necessary
              3. light therapy may be used to reduce jaundice
      b) ABO incompatibility
        (1) mother type O blood, father type A, B, or AB
        (2) fetus may have type A or B blood
        (3) blood cells of fetus hemolyze due to maternal anti-
            bodies present in mother's blood against A or B type
            blood
        (4) can occur in firstborn, does not increase in severity
            with subsequent pregnancies
        (5) disease varies in severity but is usually less severe
            than RH
        (6) higher incidence in black infants
        (7) management
           (a) every type A or B infant born to group O mother
               should have a Coombs test, hematocrit, blood
               smear and bilirubin level before discharge from
               hospital
           (b) light therapy may be used to reduce jaundice by
               breaking down bilirubin (infant's eyes must be
               protected)

    (c) exchange transfusion may be necessary
   c) implications for nursing care
    (1) education of prospective parents to prevent sensitization
  5. hypertensive states of pregnancy (Wingate, 1978)
   a) classification
    (1) preeclampsia and eclampsia
    (2) hypertensive disease in pregnancy
     (a) acute renal disease
     (b) chronic hypertensive vascular disease (see p. 100)
     (c) superimposed preeclampsia or eclampsia
   b) preeclampsia and eclampsia
    (1) occurs only in pregnancy, usually after twentieth week
     (a) may occur before the twentieth week when trophoblastic disease is present
    (2) higher incidence in
     (a) primigravidas
     (b) adolescents
     (c) women over 30
     (d) low socioeconomic groups
     (e) diabetic women
     (f) women with chronic hypertension
     (g) women with trophoblastic molar disease
    (3) etiology is unknown
    (4) characteristics of the condition are hypertension, edema, and/or proteinuria
    (5) mechanisms
     (a) increased vascular reactivity resulting in widespread vasospasm and vasoconstriction
     (b) blood supply to organs may be reduced
      1. organs most seriously affected are brain, kidney, liver and placenta
     (c) alteration in fluid and sodium retention
     (d) leakage of plasma protein into the urine from the glomerular membranes of the kidney
    (6) symptoms of mild preeclampsia
     (a) a sudden onset of weight gain of two or more pounds a week
     (b) a sustained rise in BP of 30 mm or more systolic and, 15 mm or more diastolic over the prepregnancy or early pregnancy levels. BP in mild preeclampsia will remain below 160/110
     (c) urinary protein is less than 5 g/24 hr
     (d) edema may be absent or mild
    (7) severe preeclampsia
     (a) BP rises 60/30 mm Hg or more above early pregnancy or prepregnancy levels. BP will rise above 160/110
     (b) urinary protein excretion will rise above 5 g in 24 hours

       (c) urinary output will decrease to 500 ml or less in 24 hours (oliguria)

       (d) massive generalized or pulmonary edema may occur

       (e) epigastric pain and cerebral or visual disturbances may be present (headache, blurring of vision, spots and double vision, hyperreflexia)

(8) effect of preeclampsia on fetal development

       (a) mild preeclampsia will usually not adversely affect the fetus

       (b) as preeclampsia becomes more severe the decrease in placental perfusion of nutrients and oxygen may cause fetal hypoxia and an inadequate nutritional intake

       (c) monitoring of fetal development includes

          1. measurement of fundal height and FH rate

          2. ultrasonic cephalometry

          3. urinary estrial levels

          4. stress and nonstress fetal heart monitoring

(9) treatment of preeclampsia

       (a) the treatment of this condition has changed radically over the past few years and is still a subject of controversy. The goal of treatment is to prevent the occurrence of eclampsia and cerebrovascular and cardiovascular problems and to deliver an infant in good condition

       (b) the former treatment of preeclampsia placed an emphasis on the use of diuretics and low salt diets. Recent research indicates that this type of therapy may lead to

          1. maternal electrolyte imbalance due to depletion of sodium and potassium

          2. hemorrhagic pancreatitis

          3. infants may develop electrolyte imbalance

          4. placental blood flow may be reduced because of a decrease in the circulating blood volume

c) current management of mild preeclampsia includes

    (1) management on an ambulatory basis

    (2) ample protein diet without restriction of salt or fluids (excessive salt intake should be avoided)

    (3) frequent rest periods in lateral recumbent position

    (4) avoid fatigue

    (5) reduce stress

       (a) assist women through support and counselling to cope with stress factors

    (6) education regarding pregnancy in general and about the management of the present condition. Signs of change in the state of the condition must be carefully taught

    (7) frequent and comprehensive prenatal care and monitoring must be provided

    d) if condition progresses to severe preeclampsia, client must be hospitalized
      (1) complete bed rest in lateral recumbent position (increases glomerular filtration and promotes diuresis)
      (2) diuretics may be prescribed for a short period of time with strict control of electrolytes, if bed rest is not effective and if pulmonary edema occurs
      (3) the use of antihypertensive drugs is controversial but is used if severe hypertension persists in order to prevent cerebrovascular accidents
      (4) termination of the pregnancy is the only really effective treatment for severe preeclampsia when the response to treatment is unsatisfactory or the pregnancy is near term. Induction of labor or cesarean section may be used
    e) nursing care in preeclampsia
      (1) assessment
        (a) nutritional status and dietary pattern
        (b) knowledge about what occurs during pregnancy
        (c) activity and rest patterns
        (d) frequent regular monitoring of vital signs, FH, weight gain, presence of significant symptoms or changes
        (e) possible family and environmental stressors
      (2) intervention
        (a) educate client for self-management of own care including current condition, course of pregnancy, nutrition, rest, etc.
        (b) report any significant change to physician
        (c) assist client to cope with identified stressors
        (d) make referrals to other agencies when client needs further assistance
    f) eclampsia
      (1) symptoms
        (a) increase in severity of symptoms of preeclampsia
          1. blood pressure 180/110
          2. albumin 4+
          3. oliguria or anuria
          4. increased neurological involvement
          5. coma and convulsions
      (2) management
        (a) most eclampsia can be prevented by rigorous treatment of preeclampsia
        (b) hospitalization and bed rest
        (c) sedation
          1. barbiturates and tranquilizers are used
        (d) magnesium sulfate blocks neuromuscular transmissions and depresses the CNS
          1. magnesium sulfate is usually given as a 50% solution: 10 g administered in two 10 ml doses by deep IM injection as initial dose, followed

by 5 g, dose IM q 4 hr. As magnesium sulfate
is painful, it should be given deep in the gluteal
muscle by deep Z track and the site massaged
2. has been given by IV slow infusion in 10-20%
solution
3. magnesium sulfate is excreted mainly by kidneys and toxic levels may lead to cardiore-
spiratory arrest
4. blood levels should be monitored. Therapeutic level range of drug is 2.5-7.5 mEq/l.
Toxic level is 12-14 mEq/l
5. Signs of hypermagnesium may appear at 4
mEq/l. Signs include
a. thirst
b. flushing and feelings of heat
c. sweating
d. depression of reflexes
e. flaccidity
f. extreme signs include circulatory collapse,
CNS depression, and respiratory paralysis
(1.) CNS depression signs include anxiety
changing to drowsiness and coma
6. medication should be withheld and doctor notified if
a. respirations drop below 12/min
b. knee jerk reflex is absent
c. urinary output drops below 30 ml/hr during
IV infusions or 120 ml q 4 hr when IM dosage is administered
7. calcium gluconate is used as an antidote to
magnesium sulfate in severe CNS depression
(e) medications to promote vasodilation and lower
blood pressure may be used
(f) high protein diet
(g) intake and output recorded
(h) parenteral fluid therapy - prevents acidosis
(i) termination of pregnancy if not able to control
progression of symptoms
(3) all symptoms usually disappear 2-4 weeks after delivery unless chronic hypertension or kidney damage
occurs
(4) implications for nursing process
(a) severe restriction of all stimuli
1. restrict visitors
2. darkened quiet room
3. plan nursing care to cause least amount of dis-
turbance to patient
(b) protect against injury during convulsions
1. side rails used with padding to prevent injury
2. padded tongue blade on hand to prevent injury
to tongue. Do not force into clenched teeth

(c) constant observation
1. blood pressure, pulse, and respiration taken frequently
2. neurological status constantly monitored
3. kidney function checked by measuring urinary output and intake
(d) client and family will need additional support and information to help them cope with the crisis as eclampsia is life-threatening

6. diabetes (Brown, 1978)
a) during pregnancy, hormonal products are produced in the mother's body that act as antagonists to maternal insulin. Human placental lactogen is the most important of these hormones which decrease the amount of available maternal insulin. In response to this the rate of maternal insulin secretion increases. The rate of insulin production also increases to meet the increased level of blood glucose needed to meet fetal energy requirements.
b) if the maternal pancreas cannot secrete enough insulin CHO intolerance and gestational diabetes may develop
c) classes of diabetes in pregnancy (White classification system)
   (1) class A (gestational): asymptomatic abnormal glucose tolerance test, normal fasting blood sugar, no insulin requirement. Glucose tolerance test usually returns to normal following delivery. A small percentage (25%) may develop diabetes within 5.5 years. May be managed on diet restrictions, no other therapy needed
   (2) class B: diabetes with onset after age 20, duration less than 10 years. No sign of vascular disease
   (3) class C: onset of diabetes ages 10-19; duration 10-19 years. No signs of vascular disease
   (4) class D: onset of diabetes before age 10; duration 20 years or more. Vascular lesion such as benign retinopathy, hypertension calcified arteries in lower extremities
   (5) class E: pelvic arteries calcification
   (6) class F: diabetic nephropathy
   (7) class R: proliferative retinopathy
   (8) class G: frequent pregnancy failures
   (9) class H: cardiopathy
d) rate of occurrence
   (1) gestational diabetes: 1-2% of pregnancies
   (2) pregestational diabetes: 0.1-0.2% of pregnancies
e) women at risk
   (1) previous oversized babies (over 4000 g - 9 lbs)
   (2) previous unexplained perinatal deaths or congenital anomalies

      (3) habitual abortions
      (4) polyhydramnios
      (5) familial diabetes particularly in siblings and parents
      (6) glycosuria (must differentiate between lactosuria and renal glycosuria)
      (7) obesity that is over 20% of ideal weight
      (8) history of preeclampsia
      (9) chronic vaginal moniliasis
    (10) retinopathy or neurosensory disorders

f) diagnosis
      (1) all women at risk should have a glucose tolerance test
      (2) some physicians recommend that all gravidas above age 25 should be screened with a 1-hour glucose tolerance test. If true blood glucose levels are 130 mg/100 or more then a full glucose tolerance test should be performed
      (3) women with pregestational diabetes are given tests with fasting blood sugars

g) influence of diabetes on pregnancy
      (1) fetus may respond to increased and varying levels of blood glucose with fetal pancreatic beta cell hyperplasia and fetal hyperinsulinism
      (2) elevated fetal insulin production may cause increased fetal body fat and organ weights (oversized infants)
      (3) synthesis of pulmonary surfactant may be delayed increasing the risk of respiratory distress syndrome
      (4) after delivery the hypertrophied pancreas of the body is still secreting increased amounts of insulin but the mother's blood glucose is no longer supplying glucose. This may cause severe neonatal hypoglycemia
      (5) episodes of hypoglycemia in utero may be a factor in causing an increased rate of stillbirths
      (6) increased incidence of hypocalcemia of neonate
      (7) there is an increased incidence of preeclampsia
      (8) increased incidence of difficult labor and hydramnios
      (9) increased incidence of congenital malformations
    (10) increased rate of perinatal mortality
    (11) increased prematurity and RDS in neonates

h) influence of pregnancy on diabetes
      (1) first 20 weeks of gestation
         (a) output of insulin antagonist hormones is small
         (b) there may be a modest decrease in maternal insulin requirements
         (c) women maintained on their prepregnancy doses of insulin may experience hypoglycemic episodes
      (2) at 20 weeks gestation insulin requirements increase due to increased placental mass and increased secretion of insulin antagonists into maternal blood
         (a) danger of hyperglycemia and acidosis. Insulin needs decrease during labor

(3) immediately following delivery diabetic becomes extremely insulin sensitive and must be carefully monitored. Insulin need may drop dramatically during first 2 or 3 days following delivery. Normal insulin needs usually develop in 6 weeks postpartum

(4) long-term influence of pregnancy on diabetes is not clearly known. In clients with advanced classifications and the presence of advanced retinopathy or nephropathy some physicians may recommend abortion

i) management

  (1) gestational diabetes can usually be managed by diet control

    (a) weight gain of 25 lbs should be goal

    (b) avoidance of sweets

    (c) placed on 1800-2200 calorie diabetic diet

    (d) the obese diabetic should not diet during pregnancy

    (e) sufficient calories must be taken to prevent ketonemia and ketonuria

    (f) blood glucose level is monitored by regular fasting and 2-hour postprandial blood glucose levels. If fasting blood glucose rises over normal levels insulin may be needed

  (2) diabetic pregnancy

    (a) establishment of accurate (EDC) estimated date of confinement through menstrual history, fundal height, quickening, and ultrasonic measurement of crown-rump length or serial fetal biparietal diameter

    (b) dietary management: weight gain goal is 25 lbs; 30/35 cal/kg of ideal body weight per day including 100-125 g protein, 200-250 g CHO, 70-80 g fat. Avoidance of concentrated sweets

    (c) careful evaluation of renal function and examination of fundi

    (d) baseline blood pressures are taken with frequent follow-up monitoring

    (e) insulin management

      1. goal: to keep blood glucose levels within normal range

      2. method to reach goal

        a. adherence to prescribed diet

        b. careful regulation of activity

        c. correlation between blood glucose level and urine glucose level is low

        d. a glucose oxidose impregnated finger stick can be used by the patient to determine blood levels. Fasting blood sugars are performed regularly by physician

5. careful monitoring of insulin dosage is essential throughout the pregnancy. Physician may prescribe split doses of combined intermediate and short-acting insulins
6. mother usually seen weekly
7. renal function is regularly assessed. Periodic 24-hour urines are done for total protein and creatinine clearance
8. fetal monitoring at 34 weeks becomes intensive
   a. stress and nonstress testing and fetal movement count. A significant drop in the number of fetal movements may necessitate immediate hospitalization
   b. oxytocin challenge test monitors fetal status
   c. urinary estriol can be monitored
   d. fetal maturity may be assessed by measuring amniotic fluid lecithin-sphingomyelin ratio
9. delivery is timed to prevent fetal injury; between 36-38 weeks is a risk point for the fetus. Careful monitoring of fetal maturity and fetal status enables the physician to determine the optimum time for delivery
10. induction of labor is usually attempted with IV pitocin. If induction is not successful a cesarean section is performed
11. postpartum insulin dosage is usually decreased following delivery
12. diabetics may successfully breast feed their infants (caloric intake must be increased)

j) implications for nursing care
   (1) assess the level of understanding of the effect of the pregnancy on the diabetes and the diabetes on the pregnancy
   (2) assist woman in a more rigorous maintenance of balancing dietary activity and insulin requirements as infant outcome is related to maintaining appropriate insulin blood levels at all times
   (3) close and frequent monitoring of the pregnancy

7. cardiac disease (Gowda, 1978)
   a) classification (established by New York Heart Association)
      (1) class I: heart disease with no limitation of activity and no abnormal symptoms
      (2) class II: heart disease with slight limitation of activity. Comfortable at rest; ordinary activity causes symptoms of fatigue, dyspnea, palpitations, pain
      (3) class III: heart disease with marked limitation of activity. Comfortable at rest; less than ordinary activity causes symptoms
      (4) class IV: heart disease with symptoms at rest; cannot perform any activity without discomfort

b) classes I and II may deliver without too much danger.
   Classes III and IV have high mortality rates; abortion
   may be considered
c) normal physiologic cardiovascular changes during pregnancy; important to differentiate from symptoms of
   heart disease
   (1) increase in maternal cardiac output
       (a) 20-24 weeks resting cardiac output increases up
           to 40%
       (b) remains up until last 8 weeks of pregnancy when
           it begins to decrease
       (c) in last trimester cardiac output is influenced by
           posture
           1. in supine position the enlarged uterus impedes
              venous return from lower extremities and de-
              creases cardiac output
           2. lateral recumbent position decreases the im-
              pediment of venous return and helps to main-
              tain increased cardiac output
       (d) heart rate increases during pregnancy (may reach
           15 beats above normal per minute at term)
       (e) hyperventilation may occur (influenced by pro-
           gesterone)
           1. there may be incidents of paroxysmal tachy-
              cardia
       (f) a systolic murmur (grade 1-3) may develop
d) diagnosis of heart disease during pregnancy
   (1) cardiac enlargement (shown on x-ray)
   (2) diastolic murmur
   (3) systolic murmur (minimum of grade 4 intensity)
   (4) severe arrythmias
e) usual causes of maternal heart disease are congenital
   heart defects or damage caused by rheumatic fever
f) maternal risks: severe disability or mortality
   (1) pulmonary edema
   (2) heart failure
   (3) atrial fibrillation and embolization
   (4) bacterial endocarditis
g) fetal risks: depend on the severity of the maternal condition; cardiac failure may lead to perinatal mortality.
   Severe heart disease may lead to abortion or retardation of intrauterine growth
h) management
   (1) class I and II
       (a) strict supervision
       (b) prevent obesity: monitor salt intake, prevent
           anemia
       (c) physical activities restricted to avoid fatigue
       (d) adequate rest and sleep
       (e) avoid stress and exposure to infections
       (f) can usually carry to term with minimal problems

        (2) class III and IV
- (a) may need hospitalization
- (b) strict bed rest
- (c) sodium restriction
- (d) careful dietary monitoring: adequate but not excessive calories, iron and protein intake must be adequate
- (e) digitalis and thiazide diuretics
    1. can cross placental barrier
    2. careful supervision of fluid and electrolyte balance
    3. may need additional potassium
- (f) prevention of stress and infection
- (g) prophylactic antibiotics are sometimes prescribed for clients with rheumatic heart disease

        (3) labor and delivery must be carefully managed
- (a) prolonged labor avoided
- (b) cardiac monitor may be needed
- (c) danger of pulmonary edema or heart failure is present during labor, delivery and immediately postpartum
- (d) analgesia must be carefully prescribed to prevent hypotension or respiratory depression in the newborn
- (e) IV fluids must be carefully monitored to prevent circulatory overload

    i) implications for nursing care
        (1) assessment
- (a) client understanding of her condition and the influence of pregnancy on same
- (b) client ability and motivation to adhere to prescribed regime
- (c) frequent monitoring of vital signs and signs of client discomfort during rest and activity
- (d) nutritional and activity and rest patterns

        (2) intervention
- (a) assistance in maintaining prescribed regimen through teaching, counselling and referrals
- (b) teaching client to recognize signs of significant change
- (c) careful observation of any signs of change or danger, throughout the pregnancy cycle

8. hypertension in pregnancy
   - a) chronic hypertension present in the prepregnant state
   - b) hypertension only during pregnancy
   - c) in preeclampsia increase in BP usually occurs after twenty-fourth week. In hypertensive disease increase usually occurs earlier
     - (1) may drop in first two trimesters and rise again during third
     - (2) sustained BP of 140/90 is usually a sign of condition (except in cases of hydatidiform mole)

    d) risk factors include older women, family history, and obesity
    e) study of eye grounds, blood, urine chemistry and kidney function provide a more definitive diagnosis
       (1) creatinine and BUN levels are useful in determining prognosis of the pregnancy
    f) management
       (1) high protein diet with adequate calories
       (2) frequent rest periods in left lateral position to improve utero-placental and renal perfusion
       (3) clients on antihypertensive medication before pregnancy are maintained on the same medication. Dosage may need to be decreased during first and second trimester with an increase in last trimester
       (4) medications are used only if necessary as they cross the placental barrier. Careful monitoring of client on medication is necessary
       (5) monitoring of fetal well being
          (a) serial estriol
          (b) HPL determination
          (c) oxytocin challenge testing
          (d) if estriol and OCTs are normal, pregnancy is allowed to come to term. When L/S ratio indicates fetal maturity and cervix is ready, induction of labor is done
          (e) if fetal distress becomes evident induction is done even with an immature fetus
       (6) implications for nursing care
          (a) assessment
             1. observation for changes in vital signs or other significant changes
             2. nutrition, activity and rest
             3. stressors
          (b) intervention
             1. teaching and counselling regarding condition, management of treatment regimen, detection of significant change, nutrition, rest and activity
             2. assist client in identifying and coping with areas of present and potential stress
9. infections
    a) respiratory
       (1) may cause decrease of oxygen supply to fetus
       (2) tuberculosis
          (a) rate of new cases of TB has declined steadily in this county with the advent of chemotherapy. There are still, however, new cases reported each year and the incidence in poor urban areas can be significant
          (b) inactive TB may become reactivated during pregnancy

       (c) diagnosis is based on
1. history and physical
2. tuberculin skin test
3. chest x-ray for positive skin test
4. bacteriological culture of sputum

       (d) chest x-ray must be carefully weighed because of its potential hazard to fetus of radiation exposure. A protective lead shield is used to protect the fetus during the x-ray

       (e) treatment is chemotherapy
1. drug of choice is isoniazed in combination with a variety of other drugs in order to prevent drug resistance
2. other antituberculosis drugs used with isoniazed are ethambutal, streptomycin and rifampin
3. most drugs are not dangerous to fetus with exception of streptomycin which may affect the acoustic nerve
4. hospitalization is not required
5. client is instructed to carry out isolation precautions until sputum is negative for tubercle bacillus
6. congenital tuberculosis is rare but can occur
   a. neonate born to a woman with acute untreated TB must be carefully screened
7. in active, sputum-positive cases of TB, infant must be separated from mother in order to prevent spread of disease to the baby. When sputum becomes negative many doctors recommend BCG vaccine for babies born to active, sputum-positive mothers
8. mother should not breast feed in active cases
9. infant should be followed up with regular tuberculin skin testing

       (f) implications for nursing care
1. assessment
   a. client understanding of condition and its effect on pregnancy and its communicability
   b. client nutrition, activity and rest patterns
   c. client and family acceptance of condition
2. intervention
   a. teaching and counselling regarding self-management of treatment regime, diet, activity and medical aseptic measures
   b. assist client to accept condition and to accept possible separation from infant if it is necessary

   b) venereal diseases
     (1) dangerous to the neonate
       (a) syphilis: screening by VDRL or RPR tests

       1. possibility of development of congenital syph-
ilis if mother does not receive treatment during first trimester of pregnancy
   (b) gonorrhea: causes ophthalmia neonatorium if not
treated; diagnosed by cultures
       1. instillation of prophylactic eye medication in
neonate to prevent infection
  (2) antibiotics are used in treating the condition
  (a) penicillin is the drug of choice
c) herpes vaginalis
  (1) herpes virus type II: usual causative organism; transmitted venereally
  (2) delivery by cesarean section because of danger to
infant from infection by the virus
   (a) may seriously affect the CNS, visceral organ and
cardio-respiratory organs of the infant
  (3) infant is isolated
  (4) herpes has been treated with photosensitive proflavin
(red dye) followed by exposure to fluorescent light for
15 minutes. While this treatment has been found to
alleviate symptoms, viral particles may enter the
cells without killing the cells and may act as carcino-
gens. This therapy has presently been discontinued
  (5) there is no cure at present
  (6) if membranes have ruptured baby is at risk for development of disease even if a cesarean section is
performed
  (7) implications for nursing care
   (a) client must be educated as to the danger that the
infection poses to the newborn
   (b) immediate reporting to physician if membranes
rupture
   (c) client counselled to have frequent follow-up pap
smears
d) monilia (vaginal infection caused by candida albicans)
  (1) if infection is present at delivery, neonate may develop
thrush - treated with mycostatin and gentian violet
e) urinary infections
  (1) pyelonephritis of pregnancy is related to dilation of
the ureters and urinary stasis. Early treatment of
any urinary infection with appropriate antibiotic or
urinary antiseptic is important in the prevention of
the development of pyelonephritis
  (2) pyelonephritis is treated with hospitalization, bed rest
in semi-Fowlers position, IV fluids and ampicillin
therapy
  (3) when other urinary infections such as cystitis are
being treated sulfonomides should not be used in last
few weeks of pregnancy because of the danger of hyperbilirubinemia in the newborn

f) cytomegalovirus is found commonly in vagina during pregnancy
  (1) may be asymptomatic in mother
  (2) can cross placenta to infect fetus. May cause abortion, microcephaly, blindness, perceptual disorders and other conditions associated with retardation of intrauterine growth
  (3) may cause brain damage to newborn after delivery if infection is transmitted
  (4) diagnosis of disease
    (a) tissue cultures from urine
    (b) complement fixation antibody test
  (5) no treatment is available

g) toxoplasmosis: infection by a protozoan which is ingested as cysts in undercooked meat, or is acquired through handling the excreta of an infected cat
  (1) usually mild in the adult; resembles infectious mononucleosis
  (2) fetus has a 40% chance of developing the disease (death rate 10-15%)
    (a) can cause chorioretinitus, a severe CNS syndrome with encephalitis, carditis and other serious conditions
  (3) diagnosis made by a positive Sabin-Feldman dye test which indicates a recent or active infection
  (4) treatment
    (a) if disease is severe in the mother she can be treated with sulfadiazine, pyremethamine, and folinic acid
    (b) treatment does not prevent fetal disease
    (c) abortion may be desired by the parents because of the high probability of severe damage to the fetus
  (5) nursing implications: counsel pregnant women not to eat raw or undercooked meat or to handle cat litter

h) rubella infection in the mother carries a very severe danger to the fetus. Infection in the first 8 weeks carries greatest risk. In the third trimester there are no risks
  (1) causes abortions, growth retardation, blindness, deafness, mental retardation and other serious problems
  (2) women who have not had the disease in childhood should be immunized before they become pregnant
  (3) a test for antibodies can indicate whether or not a woman has had the disease
  (4) nursing implications include preventative education regarding immunization against the disease in childhood. Women who contract the disease when they are pregnant will need support if they contemplate an abortion

# CHAPTER 9

## DRUGS USED DURING THE PRENATAL PERIOD

A.  All drugs used during pregnancy should be prescribed with extreme caution because of possible teratogenic effects (congenital malformations)

1. the nurse should counsel the patient about the possible effects of any drug prescribed and should caution her about the use of any over-the-counter drug or drugs that have not been prescribed
2. since November, 1980, a revised food and drug labeling program has been in effect; all prescription drugs that have a potential for harm to the fetus or are absorbed systemically must be categorized according to level of risk to fetus
   a) category A: controlled studies in women fail to demonstrate a risk to the fetus in the first trimester (and there is no evidence of a risk in later trimesters), and the possibility of fetal harm appears remote
   b) category B: either animal reproduction studies have not demonstrated a fetal risk but there are no controlled studies in pregnant women, or animal reproduction studies have shown adverse effect (other than a decrease in fertility) that was not confirmed in controlled studies in women in the first trimester (and there is no evidence of risk in later trimesters)
   c) category C: either studies in animals have revealed adverse effects on the fetus (teratogenic or embryocidal effects or other) and there are no controlled studies in women, or studies in women and animals are not available. Drugs should be given only if the potential benefit justifies the potential risk to the fetus
   d) category D: there is a positive evidence of human fetal risk, but the benefits from use in pregnant women may be acceptable despite the risk (e.g., if the drug is needed in a life-threatening situation for a serious disease for which safer drugs cannot be used or are ineffective). There is an appropriate statement in "warnings" section of the labeling
   e) category X: studies in animals or human beings have demonstrated fetal abnormalities or there is evidence

105

of fetal risk based on human experience, or both, and
the risk of the use of the drug in pregnant women clearly
outweighs any possible benefit. The drug is contraindicated in women who are or may become pregnant. There
is an appropriate statement in the "contraindications"
section of the labeling

Also included in the new labeling requirements is a
drug's known effects on reproduction and any nonterato-
genic adverse effects, such as narcotic withdrawal symptoms in the newborn or hypoglycemia in the fetus attributed to the mother's use of the drug

B. Changes in maternal physiology that affect drug action
   1. drug absorption: believed to be similar to the nonpregnant
      state
   2. serum albumin has lower concentration levels because of
      increase in volume of plasma thus decreasing albumin-
      binding capacity of the drug resulting in more "free" drug
      for placental transfer
   3. increase in amounts of circulating steroid hormones influ-
      ences the metabolism of drugs in the liver
      a) hepatic blood flow is not increased
      b) some bile stasis may occur as pregnancy advances; this
         may delay degradation of drugs
   4. increased renal perfusion and glomerular filtration may in-
      crease the speed of drug excretion

C. The role of the placenta
   1. drugs are transferred across the placenta primarily by
      simple diffusion
   2. drug transfer is greater during late pregnancy
   3. any drug in sufficient concentration will eventually cross
      the placenta (Rayburn and Zuspan, 1980)
   4. some drugs may act on fetoplacental unit and reduce pla-
      cental blood flow or interfere with the active transport or
      other nutritive functions of the placenta

D. Drug effects on the fetus
   1. some drugs crossing the placental barrier usually reach
      fetal levels which correspond to 50-100% of maternal se-
      rum concentrations
   2. total drug exposure of the fetus is more important than rate
      of placental transfer
   3. chronic exposure to a drug may influence fetal cell growth
   4. some drugs have higher affinity for specific target areas,
      for example
      a) heart - digoxin
      b) skeleton - tetracycline, warfarin
      c) red blood cells - sulfonamides

        d) otic nerve - streptomycin
        e) platelets - aspirin
    5. pharmodynamic effects of drugs may be more pronounced in the fetus than the mother because the activity and concentration of some liver enzymes and rate of some enzymatic reactions are probably less in the fetus
    6. excretion of most drugs is slower in the fetus
        a) excretion takes place by
           (1) simple diffusion through placenta
           (2) fetal kidneys into amniotic fluid
               (a) amniotic fluid can be swallowed by fetus
    7. drug treatment of the fetus
        a) the drug treatment of various fetal complications is being investigated. The risks and benefits of such treatment is unclear
        b) drug administration takes place by
           (1) passive transplacental route
           (2) direct intra-amniotic instillation

E.    Drugs used in normal pregnancy
    1. before drugs are used, nonpharmacological measures should be attempted to relieve discomforts. The woman should be warned against using over-the-counter drugs. Before administering a prescribed drug, the nurse should check the dosage, adverse effects and the possibility of a teratogenic effect on the fetus
    2. antacids
        a) should be avoided during first trimester when possible
        b) during late pregnancy because of slight relaxation of the cardiac sphincter and pressure of enlarging uterus there may be some regurgitation of stomach acid into the esophagus causing heartburn. An antacid may be prescribed by the physician
           (1) the patient should be warned about taking extra doses
               (a) large quantities of calcium carbonate may cause an increase in the secretion of stomach acid
               (b) sodium bicarbonates should be avoided during pregnancy
                   1. high sodium content
                   2. systemic absorption
                   3. produces gaseous $CO_2$ in the stomach
               (c) large doses of magnesium trisilate may damage fetal kidneys
               (d) magnesium hydroxide may damage fetal neurologic and neuromuscular systems
    3. antiemetics
        a) nausea and vomiting is a common complaint during the first trimester. All medication must be by prescription and should be used cautiously
           (1) Bendectin: two tablets at bedtime, additional tablet in morning if necessary

         (a) may cause dry mouth, drowsiness, rash, nervousness, constipation, anorexia

    (2) Tigan: 250 mg p.o. t.i.d. or q.i.d.; 200 mg rectally, t.i.d. or q.i.d. or 200 mg IM, t.i.d. or q.i.d.

         (a) suppository should not be given to benzocaine-sensitive individuals

         (b) may cause drowsiness, skin reactions. Rarely it may cause dizziness, depression, diarrhea, headache, jaundice, muscle cramps

4. laxatives
   a) constipation may occur during pregnancy, the physician may order a laxative or stool softener
   b) the following should NOT be used during pregnancy
      (1) liquid petroleum, for example, mineral oil: blocks absorption of fat soluble vitamins
      (2) danthron: absorbed systematically
      (3) castor oil: too severe for pregnancy
      (4) Clysodrast: may be hepatotoxic

5. analgesics
   a) pain may be experienced during pregnancy. It is usually the result of low back pain, sciatic, headache or muscle cramps
   b) should be used sparingly. All analgesics should be avoided during organogenesis - may have teratogenic effect
   c) acetaminophen: 325 mg, one or two tablets t.i.d. or q.i.d.
      (1) large, frequent doses may cause liver damage
      (2) sensitivity occurs on rare occasions, drug should be stopped
   d) aspirin: 325 mg, one or two tablets q 4 hr, p.r.n.
      (1) affects clotting time, may cause ringing in ears, gastric irritation, sweating, drowsiness, thirst
      (2) fetal hazards include
         (a) teratogenic effects
         (b) GI bleeding
         (c) hemorrhage at birth
         (d) salicylate poisoning of newborn
      (3) should be avoided during organogenesis and late in pregnancy to prevent hemorrhagic disorders during delivery
   e) Darvon: safe use in pregnancy not established

6. sedatives
   a) restlessness and difficulty in sleeping may occur in the last trimester
   b) the woman should be warned to avoid nonprescription drugs
   c) barbiturates taken near delivery may have adverse effects on neonate and analgesics or anesthetics given during delivery may be potentiated by sedatives

    7. vitamins and minerals
      a) poor nutrition increases the risk during pregnancy
      b) vitamins and minerals may be given routinely, the woman should be cautioned against supplementing the prescribed vitamin therapy
      c) high doses of vitamins A and D have been associated with fetal anomalies
      d) iron: difficult to obtain necessary iron from diet, therefore a supplement is usually prescribed
        (1) may cause gastric irritation
        (2) may cause diarrhea or constipation
        (3) causes dark stools
        (4) ferrous gluconate may enhance teratogenic effect of aspirin

F. Drugs used in high risk pregnancies
    1. infections
      a) a variety of antibiotic agents may be prescribed
      b) each drug should be checked for possible teratogenic effects as well as maternal effects or to make sure they are not contraindicated during pregnancy
    2. thromboembolic problems
      a) heparin: appears to be safe during pregnancy
        (1) dosage varies according to patient status and laboratory findings
        (2) may be given IV or subcutaneously
        (3) clotting time should be checked before administering
        (4) patient should be checked for signs of bleeding
        (5) patient should be warned about taking over-the-counter drugs especially those containing aspirin
      b) coumarin derivatives: has teratogenic and long-lasting effects but has been used without adverse effects from 14-36 weeks of gestation (Merrill and Verberg, 1976)
        (1) coumarin derivatives interact with many other drugs
        (2) dosage must be carefully and individually prescribed because the major adverse effect is overdose
          (a) patient should be followed with frequent test of prothrombin time
          (b) prothrombin time should be checked before administering
    3. cardiovascular problems
      a) cardiac glycosides (i.e., digoxin and digitoxin) increase force of myocardial contractions
        (1) drug used and dosage are individually prescribed
        (2) close observation is essential
        (3) lab experiments indicate these drugs cross the placental barrier; however, usually no adverse effects are noted in the human infant
          (a) it is important to monitor the newborn for signs of toxicity

b) hypertensive conditions: chronic or pregnancy induced
  (1) preeclampsia: new information has made the use of diuretics obsolete in the treatment of this condition
  (2) Inderal: dose varies
    (a) may lead to small placenta and growth retardation
    (b) may cause postnatal bradycardia and hypoglycemia in infant
    (c) may reduce contractibility of uterus
    (d) the variety of effects on many of the body systems mandate this drug be used cautiously during pregnancy
  (3) reserpine (many trade names): dose varies
    (a) may cause postural hypotension, bradycardia, fatigue, sedation, depression, lethargy, headache and dizziness
    (b) anesthetics and stress of labor may potentiate hypotensive effect
    (c) nasal congestion in the neonate is also a side effect, therefore, nursery personnel should be notified to observe for respiratory difficulties
  (4) Aldomet: used in moderate to severe hypertension
    (a) does not appear to affect blood flow to uterus and kidney and is being used during pregnancy
    (b) adverse effects include sedation, depression, sodium retention, dizziness and weakness
    (c) may change Coombs reaction to positive
  (5) diuretics: still used to treat hypertension not related to pregnancy; however, beneficial risks must be weighed when prescribing drugs
    (a) thiazides and furosemide are drugs of choice during pregnancy
    (b) thiazides include such drugs as Diuril, Esidrix and HydroDIURIL among others
      1. dose varies according to drug given and individual status
      2. may cause electrolyte imbalance
      3. may have adverse effects on neonatal fluid balance
      4. thrombocytopenia and elevated bilirubin levels have been observed in newborns

(c) furosemide (Lasix) has caused fetal abnormalities when taken during organogenesis. Used only in hypertensive crisis or pulmonary edema for short period only
1. contraindicated if patient is allergic to sulfonamides
2. may cause electrolyte imbalance
3. potentiates antihypertensive drugs
(6) magnesium sulfate
(a) used as a sedative and anticonvulsant
1. causes vasodilation and therefore lowers blood pressure
(b) cannot be given to a woman who is digitalized
(c) magnesium sulfate should not be given in repeated doses unless reflexes and respiratory rate are checked
1. depresses reflexes and respiration
(d) antidote is calcium; when administering magnesium sulfate an ampul of calcium gluconate should be readily available
(e) signs of intoxication include hot feeling, flushing, thirst, sweating, depressed reflexes, hypotension and flaccidity
(f) may lead to CNS depression, respiratory depression and circulatory collapse

Table 1: Reported Effects from Drug Exposure on the Fetus (From Rayburn and Iams, 1980)*

| Drugs | 1st Trimester Effects | 2nd and 3rd Trimester Effects |
|---|---|---|
| 1. Analgesics | | |
| Acetaminophen | None known | None known |
| Narcotics | None known | Depression, withdrawal |
| Salicylates | Frequent reports – none proven (see text) | Prolonged pregnancy and labor, hemorrhage |
| 2. Anesthetics | | |
| General | ↑Anomalies, abortion | Depression |
| Local | None known | Bradycardia, seizures |
| 3. Anorexics | | |
| Amphetamines | ↑Anomalies | Irritable, poor feeding |
| Phenmetrazine | Skeletal anomalies | Unknown |
| 4. Anti-infection Agents | | |
| Aminoglycosides | Skeletal anomalies | Nephrotoxic, ototoxic |
| Cephalosporins | None known | ↓positive cultures |
| Chloramphenicol | None known | "Gray baby" syndrome (?) |
| Clindamycin | None known | Unknown |
| Erythromycin | None known | None known |
| Ethambutol | None known | None known |
| Ethionamide | ↑Anomalies | None known |
| Isoniazid | None known | None known |
| Metronidazole | ?Mutagenesis/carcinogenesis | None known |
| Penicillins | None known | ↓positive cultures |
| Rifampin | None known | None known |

| Drug | | |
|---|---|---|
| Sulfonamides | None known | Hemolytic anemia, thrombocytopenia, hyperbilirubinemia |
| Tetracyclines | Impaired bone growth | Bone growth, stained teeth (enamel hypoplasia) |
| 5. Anticoagulants | | |
|    Coumadin | Nasal hypoplasia, ophthal. abn. epiphyseal stippling | Hemorrhage, stillbirth |
|    Heparin | None known | Hemorrhage at placental site with possible stillbirth |
| 6. Anticonvulsants | | |
|    Barbiturates | Anomalies (?) | Bleeding, withdrawal |
|    Carbamazepine | ↑Anomalies | Bleeding, withdrawal |
|    Clonazepam | Facial cleft | Withdrawal, depression |
|    Ethosuximide | None known | None known |
|    Phenytoin | IURG, craniofacial abn., MR, hypoplasia of phalanges | Hemorrhage |
|    Primidone | Same as barbiturates | Hemorrhage   Depletion of vitamin K-dependent clotting factor |
|    Trimethadione | IUGR, mental retardation, facial dysmorphogenesis | Hemorrhage |
|    Valproic Acid | Unknown | Unknown |
| 7. Antiemetics | | |
|    Bendectin | None known | None known |
|    Phenothiazines | None known | None known |
| 8. Cancer Chemotherapy | | |
|    Alkylating agents | Ab, anomalies | Hypoplastic gonads, growth delay |

Table 1 (Cont.)

| Drugs | 1st Trimester Effects | 2nd and 3rd Trimester Effects |
|---|---|---|
| Antimetabolites | | |
| folic acid analogs | Ab, IUGR cranial anomalies | Hypoplastic gonads, growth delay |
| pyrimidine analogs | | |
| arabinoside | Ab | Hypoplastic gonads, growth delay |
| purine analogs | Ab | Hypoplastic gonads, growth delay |
| (cytosine, 5-FU) | | |
| Antibiotics (Actinomycin) | Ab | Hypoplastic gonads, growth delay |
| Vinca alkyloids | Ab | Hypoplastic gonads, growth delay |
| Hormones | (See #13) | Hypoplastic gonads, growth delay |
| 9. Cardiovascular Drugs | | |
| Antihypertensives | | |
| alpha-methyldopa | None known | Hemolytic anemia, ileus |
| guanethidine | None known | None known |
| hydralazine | None known | Tachycardia |
| propranolol | None known | Bradycardia, hypoglycemia, IUGR with chronic use |
| reserpine | None known | Lethargy |
| Beta-synpathomimetics | None known | Tachycardia |
| Digitalis preparations | None known | Bradycardia |
| 10. Cold and Cough Preparations | | |
| Antihistamines | None known | None known |
| Cough Suppressants | None known | None known |
| Decongestants | None known | None known |
| Expectorants | Fetal goiter | None known |

| Drug | | |
|---|---|---|
| 11. Diuretics | | |
| Furosemide | None known | Death from sudden hypoperfusion |
| Thiazides | None known | Thrombocytopenia, hypokalemia, hyperbilirubinemia, hyponatremia |
| 12. Fertility Drugs | | |
| Clomiphene | Chromosomal anomalies (?) | Unknown |
| 13. Hormones | | |
| Androgens | Masculinization–female fetus | Adrenal suppression (?) |
| Corticosteroids | Cleft in animals, not in humans | Growth delay |
| Estrogens | CV anomalies | None known |
| Progestins | Limb and cardiovascular anomalies, vacterl syndrome | None known |
| 14. Hypoglycemics | | |
| Insulin | None known | Hypoglycemia (unlikely) |
| Sulfonylureas | Anomalies | Suppressed insulin secretion |
| 15. Laxatives | | |
| Bisacodyl | None known | None known |
| Dioctyl Sodium Sulfosuccinate | None known | None known |
| Mineral Oil | ↓Vitamin Absorp. | None known |
| MOM | None known | None known |
| 16. Psychoactive Drugs | | |
| Antidepressants - tricyclics | CNS (?)/limb defects | None known |
| Benzodiazepines | Facial clefts and cardiac | Depression |
| Hydroxyzine | None known | None known |
| Meprobamate | Facial clefts | None known |
| Phenothiazines | None known | None known |
| Sedatives | None known | Depression |
| Thalidomide | Phocomelia | None known |

Table 1 (Cont.)

| Drugs | 1st Trimester Effects | 2nd and 3rd Trimester Effects |
|---|---|---|
| 17. Thyroid Drugs | | |
| Anti-thyroid | | |
| 131I | Goiter, abortion, anomalies | Goiter, airway obstruction, hypothyroid, mental retardation |
| PTU | None known | Same |
| Tapazole | Aplasia cutis | Same, aplasia cutis |
| Thyroid USP | Does not cross | None known |
| 18. Tocolytics | | |
| Alcohol | Fetal alcohol syndrome | Intoxication, hypotonia, lethargy |
| Magnesium sulfate | None known | Hypermagnesemia, respiratory depression |
| Beta-sympathomimetics | None known | Tachycardia, hypothermia, hypocalcemia, hypo-hyperglycemia |
| 19. Vaginal Preparations | | |
| Antifungal agents | None known | None known |
| Podophyllin | Mutagenesis (?) | Laryngeal polyps (?), CNS effects (?) |
| 20. Vitamins (high doses) | | |
| A | Renal anomalies | None known |
| B | None known | None known |
| C | None known | Scurvy after delivery |
| D | Mental retardation | None known |
| E | None known | None known |
| K | None known | Hemorrhage if deficiency |

*Reprinted with permission: Rayburn, W.F and Iams, J.D., Drugs During Pregnancy: Part II, Drug Effects on the Fetus, Perinatal Press, October, 1980, 4 (9).

BIBLIOGRAPHY

Allensworth, D., Price, J., and Byrne, T.: Preparenting and Prenatal Care: First Steps to High Level Wellness, Health Values, September/October, 1978.

Branson, H.: Nurses Talk About Abortion, American Journal of Nursing, January, 1972.

Brown, Z.: Diabetes in Pregnancy, J. Family and Community Health - Perinatal Health Promotion. Aspen Systems Corp., Aspen, Colo. 1978, pp. 43-55.

Clark, Ann and D'Affonso, Dyanne: Childbearing: A Nursing Perspective, F.A. Davis Co., Philadelphia, 1979.

Curtis, Frances: Observations of Unwed Pregnant Adolescents, American Journal of Nursing, January, 1974.

Dickason, E., Schult, M., and Morris, E.: Maternal and Infant Drugs and Nursing Intervention, N.Y., McGraw-Hill Book Company, 1978.

Downs, Florence: Technological Advances and the Nurse-Family Relationship, Nursing Digest, May-June, 1975.

Gowda, V.: Maternal Cardiac Diseases With Pregnancy, in: Perinatology Case Studies (L. Iffy and A. Langer, eds), Med. Exam. Publ. Co., Garden City, N.Y., 1978, pp. 230-238.

Grant, A.: Clinical Problems of Ovulation Defects, Int. J. Gynecol. Obstet. 14:123, 1976.

Gullekson, D. and Temple, A.: Maternal Drug Use During the Perinatal Period. J. Family and Community Health - Perinatal Health Promotion. Aspen Systems Corp., Aspen, Colo., 1978, pp. 31-41.

Hott, Jacqueline: The Crisis of Expectant Fatherhood, American Journal of Nursing, September, 1976.

Howard, F. and Hill, J.: Drugs in Pregnancy, Obstetrical and Gynecological Survey 34/9:643-653.

Iffy, Leslie and Langer, A., Perinatology Case Studies, Med. Exam. Publ. Co., Inc., Garden City, N.Y., 1978.

Karmel, M.: Thank You, Dr. Lamaze, J.B. Lippincott, Philadelphia, 1959.

Kaufman, Sherwin: A New Hope for the Childless Couple. Simon and Schuster, N.Y., 1970.

Keller, Christa and Copeland, Pamela: Counselling The Abortion Patient is More than Talk, American Journal of Nursing, January, 1972.

Kistner, Robert: OCs and IUDs: A Challenge to Modern GYN Care, RN, September, 1976.

Laros, Bruce, et al.: Prostaglandins, American Journal of Nursing, June, 1973.

Maternity Center Association: Preparation for Childbearing. Maternity Center, N.Y., 1971.

Meleis, Afat: Self-Concept and Family Planning, Nursing Research, May-June, 1971.

Merrill, K. and Verberg, D.: The Choice of Long-Term Anticoagulants for the Pregnant Patient, Obstetrics and Gynecology 47(6): 711, 1976.

Rayburn, W.J. and Zuspan, F.P.: Drug Use During Pregnancy: Part I, Principles of Perinatal Pharmacology, Perinatal Press, Vol. 4, No. 8, September, 1980.

Rayburn, W.F. and Iams, J.D.: Drug Use During Pregnancy: Part II, Drug Effects on the Fetus, Perinatal Press, Vol. 4, No. 9, October, 1980.

Rubin, Reva: Cognitive Style in Pregnancy, American Journal of Nursing, March, 1970.

Schenke, B. and Vorherr, N.: Non-Prescription Drugs During Pregnancy, Potential Teratogenic and Toxic Effects Upon Embryo and Fetus, The Journal of Reproductive Medicine, January, 1974.

Simpson, J.W., Lawless, R.W., and Mitchell, A.C.: Responsibility of the Obstetrician to the Fetus. II. Influence of Pre-Pregnancy Weight and Pregnancy Weight Gain on Birthweight, Obstetrics and Gynecology 45:481-487, 1975.

Tiku, J.: Trophoblastic Disease, in: Perinatology Case Studies (L. Iffy and A. Langer, eds), Med. Exam. Publ. Co., Garden City, N.Y., 1978, pp. 129-143.

White, P.: Diabetes Mellitus in Pregnancy, Clinics in Perinatology 1(2):331-347, 1974.

Wingate, M.: Preeclampsia, in: Perinatology Case Studies (L. Iffy and A. Langer, eds), Med. Exam. Publ. Co., Garden City, N.Y., 1978, pp. 413-419.

UNIT III:  THE INTRAPARTAL PERIOD

The following terminology will be useful in the understanding of this unit:

Gravida:  pregnant woman

Primigravida:  first pregnancy

Primipara:  a woman who has had one delivery beyond 20 weeks

Multipara:  a woman who has delivered two or more children

Gravida:  refers to a pregnancy of any duration

Para:  refers to previous pregnancies that have reached the period of viability, i.e.,

Gravida I Para O (GIPO) - first pregnancy

She becomes a primipara after delivery of a viable fetus whether it is alive or dead at birth.

Gravida III Para O (GIIIPO) is in her third pregnancy after two abortions - when she delivers a viable child her status will be Gravida III Para I (GIIIPI).

Past obstetrical history may be recorded as 7-2-3-6. The first digit refers to the number of full term infants that a woman has delivered.  The second digit refers to the number of prematures. The third digit refers to the number of abortions.  The fourth digit refers to the number of living children.

# CHAPTER 10

## STAGES OF LABOR AND NURSING IMPLICATIONS

Labor can be considered a contest between the forces of expulsion and the forces of resistance.

I.  POSITION AND PRESENTATION (Fig. 10.1)

### TYPES OF PRESENTATIONS

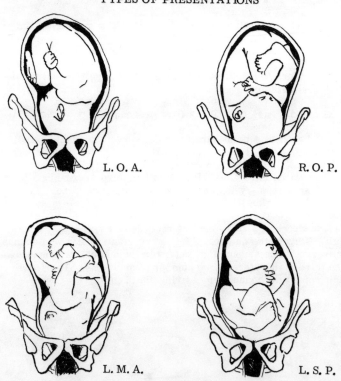

L.O.A.

R.O.P.

L.M.A.

L.S.P.

FIGURE 10.1

A.  Attitude of fetus: customary position that baby assumes in utero

  1. relationship of one part of the fetus to another
     a) arms, legs and head usually flexed
     b) fetus ovoid: conforming to uterus shape

B. Lie
   1. relationship of long axis of fetus to the long axis of mother
      can be
      a) longitudinal
      b) transverse

C. Presentation
   1. presenting part is that part of fetus which engages at inlet
      and can be felt through the cervix

D. Position
   1. determined by some arbitrarily determined point on the
      fetus to right or left side, and front or back of mother's
      pelvis
      a) position may affect the length and difficulty of the labor
         process
      b) the pelvis is divided into four regions to assist in de-
         scribing the position of the presenting part of the fetus,
         the regions are
         (1) left anterior
         (2) left posterior
         (3) right anterior
         (4) left posterior
   2. longitudinal lie: long axis of fetus parallel to long axis of
      mother
      a) cephalic positions
         (1) vertex (head sharply flexed so that vertex presents)
             (a) occiput is the point to determine this position,
                 i.e., right occiput anterior (ROA) means that the
                 occiput faces the right front of the mother's pel-
                 vis
         (2) face: (neck extended, face presents); chin (mentum)
             is point for position, i.e., left mentum anterior
             (LMA) chin faces left front of mother's pelvis
         (3) brow (siniciput) is point for position. Neck partially
             extended and brow presents
             (a) rare and difficult to deliver
             (b) frequently converts spontaneously or by version
                 to vertex or face
      b) breech positions: sacrum used as point of position
         (1) frank breech: buttocks presenting part, thighs flexed
             and legs extended
         (2) full breech: buttocks present, thighs flexed on abdo-
             men and legs flexed on thighs
         (3) footling breech: one or both feet present
         (4) right sacroposterior (RSP): sacrum faces right pos-
             terior portion of mother's pelvis

    3. transverse lie: long axis of fetus horizontal to long axis of mother
       a) shoulder presentation: scapula is the point used for determining position in a transverse lie
          (1) very rare and must be delivered by cesarean section

## II. THEORETICAL CAUSES OF LABOR

A. The precise physiological mechanisms that bring about labor are unknown. The mechanisms are complex and probably labor begins because of an interaction of factors which originate within the maternal, placental and fetal systems
    1. hormonal factors
       a) oxytocin: stimulates uterine contractions
          (1) produced by the posterior lobe of the pituitary (both fetal and maternal)
          (2) uterine sensitivity to oxytocin increases as pregnancy progresses
          (3) sensitivity of uterine muscle to oxytocin is enhanced by estrogen and inhibited by progesterone
          (4) probably oxytocin alone will not cause labor to begin, but it's presence in combination with other substances plays a role in the labor process
       b) prostaglandins: stimulate uterine contractions
          (1) widely distributed in tissues
          (2) increased uterine sensitivity to prostaglandins as pregnancy progresses
          (3) concentration increases in blood and amniotic fluid as labor progresses
          (4) there may be a relationship between the stretching of uterine muscle and production of prostaglandins
       c) change in estrogen-progesterone concentration
          (1) estrogen reaches maximum levels before the onset of labor
          (2) progesterone
             (a) blocks uterine contractions
             (b) levels decrease before labor
             (c) decrease permits estrogen influence to dominate
    2. aging of placenta
       a) degeneration of trophoblasts
       b) decrease in placental function
          (1) causes decrease in uterine blood flow
    3. uterine distension
       a) full organ tends to contract and empty itself when stretched
          (1) postulated to be a factor in premature labor with multiple pregnancies and polyhydramnios
       b) pressure on nerve endings and increased irritability of muscles may stimulate contractions

III.   MECHANISMS OF LABOR IN VERTEX PRESENTATION

A.   In order for area of least diameter of fetal head to pass
     through birth canal certain movements are necessary
     1. engagement: when largest transverse diameter of the head
        has passed through the pelvic inlet
     2. descent: gradual progressive movement throughout labor
        a) progress measured by station: relationship of vertex
           to ischial spines
           (1) station-4: head floating, freely movable
           (2) station-3-2-1: progression toward ischial spines
           (3) station 0: vertex at ischial spines - engagement
           (4) station +1 +2 +3: progression toward pelvic floor
           (5) station +4: vertex at perineum
     3. flexion: chin flexed, head tipped forward presents small-
        est head diamter to birth canal allowing further descent
     4. internal rotation: head is turned to side on the diagonal so
        that it can pass under the symphysis pubis
        a) longest diameter of fetal head aligned with largest diam-
           eter of pelvis
     5. extension: head is pushed forward through vulva V outlet
        because it offers least resistance
     6. restitution: immediately after head is born occiput rotates
        back to original position
     7. external rotation: shoulders change from transverse to
        anterior-posterior position
     8. expulsion: delivery

B.   Powers of labor include
     1. uterine contractions: the effectiveness of which are meas-
        ured by their
        a) frequency
        b) intensity
     2. voluntary abdominal muscular contractions during second
        stage of labor
     3. fetal head which acts as a battering ram to dilate cervix
        and birth canal
     4. amniotic fluid within fetal membrane which applies hydro-
        static pressure to cervix and aids in dilation

IV.   ONSET OF LABOR

A.   Premonitory signs
     1. lightening (engagement): settling of head into true pelvis
        a) usually occurs 10-14 days before labor in primigravida
        b) may not occur until labor begins in multipara
        c) increased pressure caused by descent of baby's head
           may result in
           (1) shooting pains in legs
           (2) increased vaginal discharge
           (3) frequency in urination

2. pink show
   a) discharge of mucus plug
   b) small capillaries rupture and blood mixes with mucus
3. rupture of membranes: amniotic sac (membranes) breaks causing a gush or leakage of amniotic fluid
   a) may occur prior to onset of labor, or at any stage in labor process
      (1) physician should be notified because of danger of
         (a) prolapsed cord
         (b) infection
   b) labor usually begins within 24 hours after rupture
4. early contractions may be experienced as low back pains
5. abdominal cramps
6. diarrhea
7. cervix begins to become soft and effaced and moves to an anterior position. This process is called ripening

B. Differentiation between true and false labor
   1. false labor (Braxton-Hicks contractions)
      a) contractions are irregular
      b) contractions do not increase in intensity, duration or frequency
      c) usually confined to lower segment of abdomen and groin
      d) there is no further softening or effacement of cervix
      e) no further descent of head occurs
   2. true labor
      a) contractions occur at regular intervals
      b) intervals between contractions shorten
      c) duration and intensity of contractions increase
      d) contractions usually are felt in the back and radiate to the abdomen
      e) increased cervical dilation and effacement occurs
      f) further descent of presenting part occurs

V. STAGES OF LABOR

A. First stage: starts with first true contraction and lasts until full dilation (at 10 cm) and effacement of cervix occurs
   1. duration of first stage in
      a) primigravida is usually 6-18 hours
         (1) labor is considered prolonged if first stage exceeds 20 hours
      b) multipara is usually 2-10 hours
         (1) labor is considered prolonged if first stage exceeds 14 hours
   2. characteristics of first stage of labor
      a) at onset of labor contractions usually occur every 20 to 30 minutes and are of short duration and mild intensity
         (1) each contraction has three phases
            (a) increment: increasing intensity of the contraction
            (b) acme: height of intensity of contraction
            (c) decrement: decreasing intensity of contraction

        b) intact fetal membranes increase efficiency of contraction through the mechanism of hydrostatic pressure of the fluid against the cervix

        c) contractions increase in intensity and frequency until transition stage is reached (8 cm) at which time

           (1) contractions become stronger and closer together. Sometimes they appear to be almost continuous (1 to 2 minutes apart, lasting 45 seconds)

           (2) mother may perspire profusely

           (3) mother may be nauseous and vomit

           (4) she may have a period of violent shaking and teeth chattering

           (5) there is an increase in bloody show

           (6) there may be difficulty in relaxing between contractions

        d) contractions are totally involuntary

           (1) dilation of cervix cannot be hastened by bearing down on the part of the mother

B.    Second stage: from full dilation of cervix to birth of baby

    1. duration

        a) primigravida: 30 minutes to 3 hours

        b) multipara: 5-30 minutes

    2. characteristics

        a) bloody show increased

        b) pressure on rectum causes patient to feel a desire to defecate

        c) bearing down reflex appears spontaneously

        d) voluntary abdominal musculature should be utilized to assist in bearing down

        e) perineal bulging is observed

        f) crowning: head becomes visible on perineal floor during contraction

        g) caput: head visible on perineal floor at all times

C.    Third stage: after birth of baby to birth of placenta

    1. duration: 5-10 minutes

    2. characteristics

        a) separation of placenta

           (1) gush of vaginal blood

           (2) umbilical cord descends

           (3) fundus rises in abdomen

           (4) uterus becomes firm and globular

        b) expulsion of placenta

           (1) bearing down by mother assists expulsion

           (2) Schultze mechanism: fetal side detached and expelled first

           (3) Duncan mechanism: maternal side detaches and is expelled first

D.    Fourth stage: first hour after delivery
   1. characteristics
      a) recovery from anesthesia
      b) stabilization of vital signs, bleeding and fundal muscle
         tone
         (1) may be most critical time of intrapartal period be-
             cause of increased danger of maternal hemorrhage
      c) mother may have intense emotional reactions such as
         crying to relieve tension
      d) mother usually exhausted and wants to sleep
      e) sudden severe chill may occur which is believed to be
         related to sudden change of intra-abdominal pressure or
         a nervous reaction to the childbirth experience

VI.   MANAGEMENT OF LABOR AND DELIVERY PROCESS

A.    The management of the labor and delivery process has pro-
      found immediate and long-range implications for the physical
      and emotional well being of the family unit.  Technological ad-
      vances have depersonalized the meaning of childbirth in our
      society and have also diminished the influence that parents can
      exert over the birthing process.  Parents should have an op-
      portunity to explore the implications of various childbirth man-
      agement regimes and should be allowed to make educated de-
      cisions as to the manner in which their labor and delivery will
      be conducted.
   1. areas in which decisions need to be made
      a) the place where delivery will occur
         (1) there are an increasing number of alternate birthing
             centers that can be found across the country.  These
             centers are home-like, but usually are located in or
             near a hospital
         (2) many more women choose to deliver at home.  Cau-
             tion should be advised since emergencies do arise
             unexpectedly
      b) who will be in attendance at the delivery
         (1) an increasing number of institutions allow not only
             husbands but also siblings, family members and/or
             friends to be present with the woman during labor and
             delivery
      c) when the patient is in a traditional hospital setting other
         factors need to be considered
         (1) elective induction or stimulation of labor for conveni-
             ence is contraindicated
         (2) shaving of the pubic areas
             (a) many studies indicate that shaving of the pubic
                 area does not influence the incidence of infection
             (b) many institutions have abandoned the use of the
                 pubic prep or have substituted a mini-prep of the
                 perineal area

(3) the routine use of enemas during early labor is being reevaluated
(4) use of analgesics and anesthesia
    (a) the mother should be informed of possible risks involved in the use of large doses of analgesia and anesthesia. Studies show possible risk factors to be
        1. respiratory initiation and early respiration rhythms of the newborn may be affected
        2. sucking reflex may be diminished
        3. depression of CNS of newborn may occur
        4. regional anesthesia may prevent mother from assisting in the expulsion phase, necessitating the use of forceps
        5. regional anesthesia may cause hypotension, resulting in a decrease in the oxygen supply to the fetus
(5) position during labor
    (a) most mothers are encouraged to lie on their backs
        1. causes compression of the major blood vessels by the uterus
        2. may impede progress of labor
        3. may diminish oxygen supply to fetus
    (b) most mothers are not permitted to be ambulatory
    (c) sitting, walking or assuming a side position in bed are preferable positions during labor
(6) isolation of the woman in labor
    (a) increases fear and anxiety
    (b) depersonalizes and dehumanizes the birth experience
    (c) denies the woman the opportunity to have support from people who are important to her
    (d) there is no scientific indication that the presence of someone other than health personnel during labor and delivery will adversely affect the process
(7) management of delivery
    (a) the use of lithotomy position for birth may
        1. affect blood pressure, cardiac return and pulmonary ventilation
        2. impede bearing down efforts
        3. impede placental expulsion
        4. necessitate use of episiotomy
    (b) positions that are preferable include
        1. squatting
        2. semisitting position with soles of feet firmly placed on bed
(8) immediate separation of mother and child after delivery may interfere with mother-child bonding and the successful establishment of lactation

       (9) the belief that all deliveries should take place in a hospital with a physician in attendance is open to question

          (a) nurse-midwives have been shown to effectively manage a normal labor and delivery

          (b) alternative facilities for normal deliveries are being developed by groups such as the Maternity Center of New York

      (10) use of electronic fetal monitoring

          (a) may further depersonalize care

          (b) recent studies indicate that there is an increase in infections during the perinatal period when internal monitoring devices are used

          (c) the woman cannot freely move around once the monitor is attached

B.    Nursing care during the first stage of labor

    1. admission of patient

      a) assessment

        (1) identification

        (2) vital signs (TPR, BP, FH) are monitored with increasing frequency as labor progresses

        (3) history and physical examination

          (a) history includes information essential for the management of labor and delivery

            1. obstetrical status determined, i.e., primigravida or multipara and E.D.C.

            2. history of symptoms of patient in this labor, i.e., presence of show, rupture of membranes and character and duration of contractions

            3. any allergies that are present should be recorded

            4. presence of any current or recent illness in herself or family

            5. time of ingestion of last meal

            6. plans for breast or bottle feeding

            7. when she last slept and whether she is fatigued

            8. whether or not patient feels any discomfort

            9. any special physical problems or disabilities

            10. any blood incompatibilities

            11. serological test reports

          (b) physical examination includes general and obstetrical status

            1. obstetrical examination will determine stage and progress of labor

        (4) mother's knowledge and attitudes toward labor and delivery

          (a) desires regarding management of labor and delivery

          (b) preparation for childbirth

          (c) fears and concerns

        (5) family relationships
           (a) marital status
           (b) desires regarding presence of family member or friend to be present during labor and delivery
           (c) arrangements or concerns about children at home

   b) intervention is based on the rationale that fear and anxiety increase muscular tension and lead to an increase in the perception of pain

       (1) orientation to hospital
          (a) explanation of routines
          (b) introduction of staff

       (2) provide information regarding
          (a) status of labor
          (b) what to expect as labor progresses
          (c) mechanisms to reduce pain

       (3) give medications as ordered and desired
       (4) establish a patient record
       (5) provide for draping and screening to insure client privacy
       (6) report immediately any deviations from the normal in observation of the clients general or obstetrical status

2. remainder of first stage of labor: assessment of safety, physical status and psycho-social status will determine nursing intervention

   a) level of consciousness
       (1) assessment
          (a) orientation to time and place
          (b) level of wakefulness
          (c) arousability
          (d) reaction to pain
          (e) level of concentration
          (f) time and dose of analgesia administration

       (2) intervention
          (a) protect from injury
          (b) side rails if necessary
          (c) assist in and out of bed to prevent falls

   b) environmental hazards
       (1) assessment
          (a) aseptic techniques
          (b) condition of electric equipment
          (c) temperature and air circulation of labor room

       (2) intervention
          (a) asepsis: measures must be taken to prevent the introduction of pathogens into the vaginal canal, i.e., precautions used during vaginal examination include use of sterile gloves and antiseptic preparation to cleanse perineal area

   c) physical status of mother and fetus
       (1) fetal heart

    (a) assessment
1. throughout labor the monitoring of the fetal heart rate is vital because it is an indicator of any changes in fetal condition
2. normal rate: between 120-160 beats per minute with regular rhythm
   a. rate slows at height of contraction of uterus
   b. rate increases at the end of uterine contractions
3. rate of fetal heart below 100 or above 160 with uterus at rest may indicate fetal distress
4. auscultation of fetal heart
   a. must differentiate between fetal heart and other sounds
      (1.) funic souffle: blood rushing through umbilical arteries is synchronous with fetal heart
      (2.) uterine souffle: blood going through large uterine blood vessels is synchronous with mother's pulse
   b. impediments to auscultation of FH
      (1.) maternal obesity
      (2.) pendulous abdomen
      (3.) polyhydramnios
      (4.) posterior occiput presentation
      (5.) taking of FH at height of contraction
      (6.) loud maternal souffle
   c. locations of FH
      (1.) cephalic presentations
         (a.) loudest below umbilicus
         (b.) anterior positions: FH will be heard clearly in either right or left quadrant
   d. posterior presentations: best heard at point of mother's side closest to fetal back
      (1.) breech presentation
         (a.) loudest above umbilicus
      (2.) with descent and rotation of fetus, fetal heart position changes

    (b) intervention
1. any change in fetal heart rate or rhythm that may indicate fetal distress should be reported immediately
   a. patient should be turned on side
   b. oxygen may be administered

(2) contractions
    (a) assessment
1. contractions: frequency, intensity and duration must be determined

      2. interval is considered to be from the increment of one contraction to the increment of the next

      3. one contraction following another without adequate relaxation between the two are abnormal and present danger to mother

  (b) intervention

      1. contractions less than two minutes apart or more than 90 seconds in length should be reported

      2. the nurse can assist the client in coping with discomfort by

        a. presence: laying on of hands

        b. informing her of the progress of labor and the meaning of the contractions

        c. teaching breathing and relaxation techniques

        d. giving medication as indicated and prescribed

        e. reassurance to reduce fear and anxiety

        f. applying cool cloth to forehead

        g. allowing verbalization of feelings regarding pain, discomfort and fear

        h. support attempts to follow prepared childbirth technique

        i. encouragement

(3) electronic monitoring of fetal heart and contractions

  (a) used for continuous monitoring of the frequency, intensity and duration of contractions and for continuous monitoring and recording of fetal heart rate patterns so that the FHR can be evaluated under the stress of a uterine contraction as well as during relaxation period

  (b) external monitoring: one or more sensing devices attached to woman's abdomen by straps during labor

      1. information recorded on graph paper, a continuous wave pattern is formed and represents the frequency, intensity and duration of the contraction

      2. the fetal heart rate pattern is also recorded when plotted against the labor pattern significant changes in fetal heart rate can be more accurately determined

      3. if the patient attempts to breathe abdominally for relief she may have difficulty in using the proper technique due to presence of equipment

4. straps should fit correctly, if they are too loose sensors will not pick up sounds
5. if patient moves around the sensors may become dislodged or the readings may reflect the change in position
6. if the fetus changes position, the sensors may need to be repositioned
7. it is recommended that the woman remain in the supine position. This may cause
   a. maternal hypotension - careful monitoring of maternal blood pressure is necessary
   b. back discomfort
   c. pressure on abdominal blood vessels
8. the nurse can assist the patient and her family by
   a. careful explanation of the equipment and the rationale for its use
   b. giving back rubs for discomfort

(c) internal monitoring: sensing devices are introduced directly into the uterus through the cervix
1. contraction sensor is a fluid-filled catheter that transmits changes in pressure to the monitor
2. fetal sensor is a prolonged scalp electrode placed on fetal scalp
3. internal monitoring is more comfortable for the woman, however, she may not get out of bed

(d) nursing implications
1. careful and complete explanation of procedure to mother and to any members of the family present
2. all questions should be answered
3. readjustment of external sensors whenever they become displaced
4. observation of recordings at appropriate intervals
5. give reassurance about progress of labor as well as emotional support
6. safety precautions to prevent accident from use of electric equipment should be practiced

(e) interpretation of fetal monitoring data
1. measures the fetal heart rate (FHR) and the strength of the uterine contraction (IUP)
2. baseline data

        a. measures FHR and IUP in the absence of contractions

        b. FHR evaluated every ten minutes

        c. deviations in baseline data

            (1.) bradycardia: below 120 beats per minute

            (2.) tachycardia: over 160 beats per minute

            (3.) to be considered significant, the deviation must persist through two complete contraction cycles or five minutes

            (4.) deviation should be reported to the physician

    3. periodic data

        a. measures changes in the FHR in relationship to uterine contraction

        b. any change from baseline data is termed a fluctuation

        c. a significant fluctuation is more than 15 beats a minute

        d. an increase in FHR during a contraction is called acceleration

        e. a decrease in FHR during a contraction is called deceleration

            (1.) early deceleration is a response to compression of the fetal head, it does not indicate pathology. It has an early onset in relationship to the contraction

            (2.) late deceleration: begins after the contraction is established. When persistent or it reoccurs it usually indicates fetal anoxia

                (a.) observation for the occurrence of bradycardia must take place

            (3.) variable deceleration: may occur at any time during the contraction without any uniform pattern

                (a.) may be related to partial brief cord compression

                (b.) change in the mother's position may eliminate variable deceleration

                (c.) associated with neonatal depression when severe or prolonged

  (f) significance of data

1. persistent bradycardia is an ominous sign,
   especially if it follows a contraction
   a. may indicate cord compression or separa-
      tion of placenta
   b. if turning the patient on her other side
      and administration of O$_2$ do not improve
      FHR pattern, emergency delivery, usu-
      ally cesarian section, is indicated
2. tachycardia when persistent or accompanied
   by late deceleration is an indication of fetal
   distress
3. loss of beat-to-beat variation (not induced
   by drugs such as diazepam or atropine) is
   a serious development and often indicates
   the prelude to fetal death
4. normal FHR patterns have a positive corre-
   lation to high Apgar score and low neonatal
   morbidity. An abnormal pattern, although
   related to a low Apgar score and a high neonatal morbidity, does not occur in all cases.
   More data and research needs to be done in
   order to more accurately assess the findings
   of fetal monitoring

(g) factors that may cause changes in FHR
   1. compression of vertex
   2. utero-placental insufficiency
   3. compression or occlusion of umbilical cord
   4. maternal hypotension or hypoxia
   5. contractions of unusual frequency, duration,
      or strength
   6. improper administration of oxytocics
   7. maternal position

(h) if abnormal tracings occur, the immediate nursing intervention is
   1. change patient's position from supine to side
      or from one side to another
   2. administer O$_2$ by mask (6-7 1/min)
   3. stop oxytocin administration
   4. notify physician
   5. prepare for cesarian section if pattern per-
      sists

(4) fetal blood sampling
   (a) a blood sample is obtained from the fetal scalp
       after the membranes rupture, by the physician
       1. scalp is swabbed with a disinfectant before
          puncture

(b) fetal acidosis follows fetal hypoxia
  1. some authorities believe that fetal distress can only be confirmed when FHR changes are correlated to fetal blood acidosis
(c) most infants with blood samples which read pH 7.15 or less have low Apgar scores
(d) consecutive readings of pH below 7.20 that show a continuing decrease indicate the need to assess for prompt delivery
(e) fetal acidosis may be caused by maternal respiratory alkalosis and subsequent decrease in cardiac output, which is the result of hyperventilation. Hyperventilation is usually self-limiting in the conscious adult and can be controlled by having the patient breathe into a paper bag. This probably does not have adverse effects on the fetus

(5) vital signs
  (a) assessment
    1. if TPR and BP are normal they should be monitored at systematic intervals
    2. if deviations occur more frequent monitoring should be carried out
    3. baseline pulse, temperature and blood pressure should be established
    4. blood pressure and pulse may rise slightly during active labor
    5. deviations in pulse and BP should be evaluated in relation to baseline values for each client
  (b) intervention
    1. a rise in TPR may indicate dehydration or infection and should be reported immediately
    2. a sustained rise or fall of 15 mg or more in systolic or diastolic should be reported
      a. a rise in BP may indicate toxemia
      b. a fall in BP may indicate hemorrhage, shock or reaction to drugs
        (1.) an increase in pulse rate may be the first sign of hemorrhage

(6) vaginal discharge
  (a) assessment
    1. type, amount and character of bleeding
    2. time of occurrence, amount, and character of amniotic fluid discharge
  (b) intervention

    1. differentiate between bloody show and hemorrhage

    2. if hemorrhage is suspected save all linen to evaluate blood loss and monitor vital signs

    3. bloody show increases in amount as labor progresses

    4. suspected hemorrhage should be reported immediately

    5. if head is not engaged when membranes rupture careful supervision and bedrest is indicated because of danger of prolapse of the cord

    6. after rupture of membranes fetal heart should be checked and fluid inspected for signs of meconium

    7. meconium stained fluid in a vertex presentation should be reported immediately as it presents a hazard to the fetus

    8. perineal care should be given frequently as indicated

    9. perineal pads should not be used, padding should be placed on bed

  10. aseptic technique should be utilized during all examinations

(7) contour and size of abdomen

  (a) assessment

    1. abnormal bulges or ridges

    2. check for bladder distention

  (b) intervention

    1. shape of uterus indicates fetal position and changes during the process of labor

    2. abnormal bulge or ridge may indicate Bandl's Ring

    3. a full bladder may impede labor

      a. encourage voiding

      b. catheterization may be necessary

(8) comfort

  (a) assessment

    1. objective and subjective signs of client discomfort

  (b) intervention

    1. change position frequently assisting mother to find those positions which are most comfortable

    2. if possible, ambulate until membranes rupture

    3. personal hygiene attended to

      a. frequent mouth care if fluids are restricted

      b. perineal hygiene as necessary including fresh linen on bed

    4. relief of pain
      a. support, reassurance, and assistance with breathing and relaxation measures
      b. information to counteract myths and fears of labor
      c. keep informed of progress of labor
      d. back pain may be relieved by massage, pressure or cold applications to sacral area, and a change in position
      e. medication when desired, indicated and ordered

(9) nutrition
  (a) assessment
    1. dehydration
    2. edema
    3. nausea or vomiting
    4. time of last meal
  (b) intervention
    1. fluids and solids as ordered by physician
    2. peristaltic action slows at onset of labor interfering with digestive process
    3. careful monitoring of IV fluids if administered

(10) psychosocial status
  (a) assessment
    1. feelings and fears about labor
    2. knowledge and preparation for labor
    3. desire for a member of the family or close friend to be present during the labor process
    4. cultural attitude towards pain
    5. expectations of labor management including use of medications or natural childbirth
  (b) intervention
    1. encouraging verbalization of fears and expectations about labor
    2. reassurance and explanation of labor process when indicated
    3. never leaving the patient alone for other than short periods of time
    4. nonjudgmental reactions to patient's behavior during labor
    5. allowing the patient to have the person of her choice remain with her throughout labor
    6. assisting the lay person who remains with patient to provide comfort and support for patient
    7. establishing a sincere and caring relationship with the patient so that trust is established
    8. touching the patient often provides a nonverbal means of comfort and reassurance

9. use of breathing and relaxation techniques which reduce pain and tension should be introduced to patient whenever indicated
10. reassurance and encouragment that labor is progressing normally is helpful when patient becomes discouraged at length of time involved in labor process
11. respecting patient's desire for privacy and avoiding unnecessary exposure
12. keeping the patient's family informed of her progress
13. during transition period the client's psychosocial needs become intensified
    a. contractions become stronger, longer and more frequent
    b. bearing down sensations appear
    c. client may become irritable and frightened
    d. trembling of legs may occur
    e. nausea and vomiting may occur
14. the nurse may assist the client during the transition period by
    a. reassuring her that she is entering the final stage of labor and that transition is not a long period of time
    b. helping her to refrain from bearing down until full dilation occurs
       (1.) use panting-type breathing
    c. explaining the meaning of all her symptoms

C. Nursing care during the second stage and third stage of labor
   1. assessment
      a) progress of labor
         (1) perineal bulging, crowning, and caput
         (2) bearing down effort of mother
      b) continued monitoring of all vital signs including contractions and fetal heart
      c) mother's response to the change in status of labor
   2. intervention
      a) avoid precipitate delivery: patient should be brought to delivery room at proper time
      b) surgical asepsis used in delivery room to prevent infection
      c) avoid injury by proper transportation to, and positioning in, delivery room
         (1) usual delivery position is lithotomy; trend to other positions is occurring

        (a) lithotomy position if used for a prolonged period may cause increased stasis of blood in leg veins and predispose to thrombophlebitis

        (b) if lithotomy is used care should be taken that pressure is not exerted on the popliteal vein. Padding should be used to prevent pressure

      (2) preferred positions are squatting and sitting

   d) if leg muscle cramps occur the leg should be straightened and the ankle dorsi-flexed keeping knee rigid

   e) mother assisted in effective use of bearing down impulse

   f) continued encouragement and support is essential at this time through nurse-client interaction. Pressures of delivery should not interfere with relations and communications previously established between nurse and client

   g) support and encouragement as well as careful explanations of what is happening should be given to father or other person present in delivery room

   h) observation of bleeding and vital signs

   i) administration of oxytocic as ordered by physician

      (1) syntocin, pitocin and ergotamine are commonly used; may be administered IV or IM

        (a) may be ordered first after delivery of baby and again after delivery of placenta

   j) if fundal pressure is needed to deliver placenta extreme care should be used to prevent uterine inversion

D.   Immediate care of the newborn
1. establish and maintain patent airway
   a) remove mucus from nose and mouth by wiping and gentle suctioning with bulb syringe
   b) if respiration fails to begin
      (1) stimulate crying by gentle stroking
      (2) oxygen administration
      (3) resuscitation
        (a) mouth to mouth
        (b) positive pressure
   c) position baby on side to prevent aspiration
2. keep baby warm and safe
   a) baby is wrapped
   b) may be placed in a warmer or incubator
3. identification
   a) baby's footprints and mother's fingerprints are taken in delivery room and kept on baby's chart
4. care of cord
   a) after clamping, inspect for bleeding and abnormalities
      (1) three vessels should be present
   b) no dressing needed on cord stump

    5. care of eyes
      a) prophylactic treatment for ophthalmia neonatorum required by law
      b) silver nitrate 1% is installed. Latest research indicates that irrigation with normal saline or sterile water does not diminish conjunctivitis reaction to the silver nitrate. Sodium chloride may precipitate the silver nitrate (silver chloride precipitate). American Academy of Pediatrics does not recommend rinsing (Lum et al., 1980)
      c) antibiotic ointments are not recommended because of resistance of strains of organisms and possibility of sensitivity developing in infant
    6. observation
      a) Apgar scoring done at 1 and 5 minutes after birth
        (1) heart rate, respiratory effort, muscle tone, reflex irritability, and color rated from 0-2
        (2) 10 is considered a perfect score
        (3) any baby with an Apgar below 7 after 5 minutes, must be observed for abnormalities
      b) observe and inspect newborn for any abnormalities
    7. administration of vitamin K
      a) to prevent hypothrombinemia as normal flora in intestine needed for synthesis of vitamin K is not present in newborn for approximately one week
    8. baptism
      a) if there is any danger of death of the newborn many Christian parents wish to have baby baptized
        (1) notify clergy
        (2) if unavailable, nurse or doctor should baptize child

E.    Nursing care during fourth stage
    1. assessment
      a) type, amount and character of bleeding
      b) palpate for the height and firmness of fundus
      c) vital signs should be monitored frequently
      d) observe perineal area for hematomas or edema
      e) reaction to and recovery from anesthesia
      f) observe for nausea and vomiting
      g) with conscious patients ascertain subjective symptoms of
        (1) pain
        (2) dizziness
        (3) headache
      h) mother-child-father interaction
      i) urinary output and bladder distention
    2. intervention
      a) palpate uterus frequently; should remain firm and at umbilicus

    (1) if fundus relaxes or becomes boggy, gently massage until firm

    (2) if massage fails to maintain fundal tone, notify physician immediately

b) maintain airway position and patency until recovery from anesthesia

c) protect from injury
    (1) check body alignment of anesthesized patients
    (2) side rails in place

d) if bladder becomes distended
    (1) assist in voiding
    (2) catheterization if necessary

e) give analgesia if ordered or necessary

f) mouth and personal hygiene

g) emotional support
    (1) allowing her to sleep by reducing disturbances
    (2) allowing full expression of feelings with empathy shown by nurse
    (3) allowing mother and father to see and touch baby and family as soon as she is ready to facilitate bonding
        (a) report deviations from normal mother-child interaction to the postpartal nursing staff for follow-up care

# CHAPTER 11

DRUG AND ANESTHESIA ADMINISTRATION
IN THE INTRAPARTAL PERIOD

I.   RELIEF OF DISCOMFORT DURING FIRST STAGE LABOR IS
     ACCOMPLISHED THROUGH THE JUDICIOUS USE OF VARI-
     OUS TYPES OF DRUGS

A.   Pain arises from the contractions of the uterus.  Contractions
     are necessary for labor to progress and delivery of the child
     1. pharmacological relief of pain should not interfere with the
        pattern of uterine activity

B.   Pharmacological agents to relieve pain should be selected on
     an individual basis according to the needs of the woman and to
     ensure the welfare of the fetus

C.   Pharmacological agents have effects on both the mother and
     fetus

II.  DRUGS USED IN THE INTRAPARTAL PERIOD

A.   Barbiturates are classified hypnotics and are used to produce
     sleep and mild tranquilization and sedation
     1. most commonly used barbiturates include
        a) Nembutal:  50-100 mg
        b) Seconal:  0.1-0.2 g
        c) phenobarbital:  50-100 mg
     2. method of administration is usually po but may be given
        IM or IV
     3. relatively safe for both mother and child in early labor -
        may cause slowing of contractions in mother if dosage is
        excessive for the individual.  Potentiates action of nar-
        cotics and tranquilizers.  If given late in labor or in com-
        bination with narcotics may depress newborn's respira-
        tions
     4. nursing implications
        a) careful and continuous observation of patient is neces-
           sary as excessive doses may cause respiratory and/or
           circulatory depression in the mother and child
        b) side rails must be utilized in patients receiving barbi-
           turates

142

    c) heavily sedated patients are unable to communicate the progress of labor to the nurse increasing possibility of precipitate delivery

B. Analgesics are used for relief of pain usually in combination with drugs that potentiate their effect
1. commonly used narcotics
    a) meperidine hydrochloride (Demerol) 50-100 mg IM or IV
    b) morphine 8-15 mg subcutaneously
      (1) may be used if patient has an allergy to Demerol
2. rapid analgesia effect
3. are relatively safe when used carefully early in labor; may depress maternal and fetal respiration especially when used near time of delivery
4. may slow labor if used too early; when administered after cervical dilation has progressed, may accelerate process of cervical dilation and may increase relaxation of pelvic floor through its antispasmodic action
5. nursing implications
    a) careful and continuous monitoring of maternal respirations and fetal heart rate
    b) safety precautions include side rails and observation for possible nausea and vomiting which may be a side effect of drug

C. Tranquilizers
1. tranquilizers that are commonly used include
    a) Compazine: 5-25 mg
    b) Sparine: 25-100 mg
    c) Vistiral: 25-100 mg
2. causes sedation without hypnotic effect, decreases anxiety, produces muscular relaxation - decreases incidence of nausea and vomiting
3. the ability of tranquilizers to potentiate the effect of narcotics and hypnotics allows smaller dosages of these drugs to be administered
4. relatively safe for mother and baby

D. Other drugs that potentiate narcotics and hypnotics
1. Phenergan: 25-50 mg
2. Largon: 10-30 mg
    a) both drugs act to potentiate analgesics by their sedative and anti-histaminic effect and are relatively safe for mother and baby

E. Ketamine: dissociative anesthetic
1. given IV in small doses it produces profound analgesia lasting 2-5 minutes
2. large doses associated with newborn depression and loss of maternal consciousness

      3. used at time of delivery
      4. in combination with pudendal block may eliminate need for general anesthesia in low forceps delivery
      5. latest description of the drug states that its safety during pregnancy is not established and therefore is not recommended as an anesthetic for obstetrical use (PDR, 1981)

III.    IF RESPIRATORY DEPRESSION OR NARCOSIS OCCURS FROM THE ADMINISTRATION OF HYPNOTIC AND ANALGESIC DRUGS THE NARCOTIC ANTAGONISTS ARE USED

A.    Levallorphan tartrate (Lorfan) 0.3-1.2 mg IM or IV

B.    Nalorphine hydrochloride (Nalline) 5-10 mg
      1. both drugs lessen respiratory depression due to narcotic action
      2. relatively safe for mother and baby

IV.    SCOPOLAMINE 0.4-0.6 MG IS COMMONLY GIVEN IN CONJUNCTION WITH NARCOTICS TO DRY SECRETIONS AND ACT AS AN AMNESIAC AND TRANQUILIZER

A.    May cause excessive dryness of respiratory passages and extreme restlessness and agitation. May cause flushing of skin

B.    Safety precautions such as side rails and careful observation must be carried out

C.    Acts as a CNS depressant

V.    ANESTHESIA IS USED DURING SECOND AND THIRD STAGE OF LABOR

A.    General anesthesia
      1. inhalation
         a) contraindications
            (1) prematurity
            (2) fetal distress
            (3) patient with upper respiratory infection
            (4) when patient has eaten prior to administration
            (5) in multiple births
         b) types
            (1) nitrous oxide with oxygen
               (a) given with contractions; mother does not lose consciousness
               (b) anesthesia level may be deepened after delivery
            (2) cyclopropane with oxygen
               (a) highly explosive
               (b) most potent of all agents
               (c) when given with oxytocin or vasopressors may cause cardiac irregularity

        (3) methoxyflurane (Penthane)
- (a) high-potency, volatic, nonflammable ether
- (b) not irritating to respiratory tract
- (c) contraindicated with history of liver disease
- (d) associated with renal failure

  c) nursing implications
- (1) constant observation of FH rate, maternal vital signs and uterine bleeding is necessary
- (2) anesthesia may cause fetal and/or maternal respiratory distress
- (3) may slow down uterine contractions
- (4) may relax perineal musculature causing rapid expulsion of baby

  d) disadvantages
- (1) prevents mother's participation in birth and interaction with baby after birth
- (2) stops the bearing down reflex
- (3) causes neonatal depression
- (4) predisposes woman to pulmonary aspiration
  - (a) very often woman in labor has eaten
  - (b) gravid uterus may impair function of gastroesophageal junction as a result of changes in gastric position
  - (c) gravid uterus and lithotomy position increase intragastric pressure

B.   Regional anesthesia blocks transmission of painful stimuli from uterus, cervix, vagina and perineum to thalmic pain centers in brain

  1. pudendal block
- a) local anesthetic agent blocks pudendal nerve causing perineal analgesia
  - (1) used for
    - (a) spontaneous delivery
    - (b) low forceps delivery
    - (c) episiotomy
    - (d) perineal repair
- b) does not alter maternal respiration or other body functions
- c) does not affect uterine contractions but may affect bearing down reflex
- d) doesn't affect fetal respirations

  2. paracervical block
- a) rapid complete relief of uterine pain
- b) minimal maternal side effects
  - (1) no change in vaginal and perineal sensations
    - (a) does not interfere with bearing down reflex
- c) has been associated with
  - (1) fetal bradycardia and acidosis
  - (2) fetal deaths have been reported

        d) should be avoided in preterm labors or with a fetus at high risk

        e) electronic fetal monitoring is indicated with the use of paracervical block

    3. lumbar sympathetic block

        a) relief of uterine pain

        b) associated with maternal hypotension

           (1) usually minimal and can be avoided by adequate hydration and left uterine displacement

        c) little if any fetal depression

        d) not widely used

C.  Spinal anesthesia - subarachnoid block: local anesthesia injected into CSF

    1. mid-subarachnoid block

        a) most frequently used

        b) if successful will provide complete relief from perineal pain in all patients and relief of uterine pain in 90-95% of patients

        c) has no effect on maternal or fetal respirations

        d) may cause temporary drop in blood pressure or may cause severe hypotension

           (1) if blood pressure drops below 100 mm systolic, treatment to prevent shock should be initiated

    2. high spinal block: utilized for cesarean section

        a) has higher incidence and degree of hypotension

    3. low spinal block (saddle block)

        a) usually doesn't cause hypotension

    4. spinal block at any level eliminates the bearing down reflex

        a) proper preparation of patient will allow spontaneous delivery

        b) forceps easily applied because of perineal relaxation

    5. advantages of spinal block

        a) simplicity

        b) rapidity of action

        c) high success rate

        d) low incidence of maternal and fetal side effects when properly performed

    6. contraindications

        a) infection of local site

        b) central nervous system disease

        c) cephalopelvic disproportion

        d) hypovolemia: lack of sufficient fluid in blood

        e) fear of procedure

        f) deviations in normal blood pressure

    7. disadvantages

        a) maternal hypotension

        b) bearing-down reflex abolished

        c) early relaxation of perineum

        d) post-spinal maternal headache

D. Continuous caudal block: peridural analgesia produced by injection of a local anesthetic into the sacral canal with an epidural catheter in intermittent doses
   1. maternal effects are minimal
      a) may cause hypotension
   2. criteria for use
      a) patient in active labor; contractions every 3 minutes of 40 second duration
      b) engagement
      c) dilation
         (1) 5-6 cm primigravida
         (2) 4-5 cm multipara
   3. may impede progress of labor
   4. may cause central nervous system depression of fetus if large doses are administered
   5. advantages
      a) complete absence of pain and decreased anxiety
   6. disadvantages
      a) may cause maternal hypotension
      b) may prolong labor
      c) increased incidence of forceps delivery
      d) larger doses required than with subarachnoid block
   7. contraindications
      a) fetal
         (1) prematurity
         (2) postmaturity
         (3) fetal distress
         (4) breech
      b) maternal
         (1) infection at local site
         (2) central nervous system disease
         (3) hypotension
         (4) hypovolemia
         (5) fear of procedure

E. Anesthesia for cesarean section
   1. may be subarachnoid or epidural block or general anesthesia
      a) local infiltration is no longer justified unless a skilled anesthetist is unavailable (Reeder, et al., 1980)
      b) spinal anesthesia may
         (1) provide inadequate analgesia
         (2) may cause maternal hypotension
         (3) time required may delay surgery
         (4) contraindicated in some maternal conditions
      c) general anesthesia
         (1) few contraindications
         (2) method of choice when there is maternal
            (a) hypovolemia
            (b) shock
            (c) abnormal blood coagulation

              (d)  septicemia
              (e)  fear of refusal of spinal anesthesia
        (3)  disadvantages
              (a)  associated with neonatal depression
              (b)  eliminates maternal/infant contact after delivery
              (c)  places the mother at risk for pulmonary aspiration

## VI. NURSING INTERVENTION

A. The client who receives any type of analgesic or anesthetic must have continuous monitoring of
1. vital signs
2. fetal status
3. level of consciousness

B. The nurse must have knowledge of
1. types and dosage of medications used
2. complications that may occur
3. early signs and symptoms of complications
4. actions to initiate until the arrival of appropriate medical personnel when an untoward reaction occurs

C. Provide nonpharmacological nursing support for relief of pain

# CHAPTER 12

PREPARED CHILDBIRTH

I. CAUSES OF PAIN DURING CHILDBIRTH

A. First stage of labor
1. dilation of cervix
a) distension, stretching and possible tearing
2. uterine contractions
3. stretching of the lower uterine segment
4. contractions felt
a) in lower back at beginning of labor
b) with progress during labor encircles lower torso both back and abdomen
5. descriptions of discomfort vary and intensity of pain perceived is highly individualized

B. Second stage of labor
1. stretching and distension of the birth canal and perineum
a) produces severest pain
b) causes stretching, tearing and hemorrhage within the fascia, skin and subcutaneous tissues

C. Delivery
1. decrease in pain reported at time of delivery
2. sensations usually described include pressure, stretching, splitting or on occasion burning
3. pressure of presenting part causes degree of numbness in the perineum

II. EXERCISE AND BREATHING TECHNIQUES

A. Dr. Read, an English obstetrician, began the movement encouraging natural childbirth
1. the Read method of natural childbirth assumes that a normal birth is a physiological process that should not lead to extreme pain
a) Dr. Read believed that fear and anxiety about labor which is influenced by cultural conditioning is responsible for pain during labor and delivery by inducing muscular tension
b) he further believed that this fear, tension, pain syndrome could be alleviated through education and that

proper use of the body could facilitate labor
2. the Read method consists of
    a) education about pregnancy and childbirth to dispel fears and misapprehensions
    b) exercises to strengthen and increase flexibility of muscles used in labor
       (1) pelvic rocking
       (2) tailor sitting
       (3) squatting and kneeling
    c) methods of completely relaxing body musculature
    d) breathing used throughout labor
       (1) slow abdominal breathing during the first stage. Abdomen is raised during contractions to allow the uterus to rise without pressure
       (2) during second stage of labor diaphragmatic breathing is used to assist in expulsion
       (3) moderate panting is used during delivery of head
    e) proper use of abdominal and perineal muscles during bearing down phase of labor

B.    Psycho-prophylactic method of childbirth (Lamaze Method)
    1. Dr. Lamaze was a French obstetrician who became interested in the Russian use of Pavlov's stimulus response theory to decondition women in labor to the fear-tension-pain syndrome
    2. Dr. Lamaze modified the Russian method and introduced it to the Western world
    3. the Lamaze method consists of
       a) education for childbirth to dispel fears and misapprehensions
       b) methods for achieving relaxation of body musculature
       c) conditioning for labor and delivery, through development of consciously controlled activity which displaces pain sensations of contractions in the brain
          (1) controlled variations of breathing techniques or patterns for each stage of labor
          (2) massage and counterpressure
    4. positioning is used to assist in increasing maternal comfort
    5. exercises similar to Read method to strengthen pelvic musculature

C.    Eclectic approaches
    1. increasingly prepared childbirth educators have been departing from the rigidity involved in using a particular method. Approaches to prepared childbirth are eclectic in nature and draw from various theoretical frameworks
    2. the management of the labor is the responsibility of the laboring woman and the coach. They will select from the available techniques those measures which provide the most comfort and assistance

a) objective of the techniques used are to reduce perception of painful stimuli and discomfort and to assist the birth process through active participation, relaxation of the body musculature and the correct use of the muscles of expulsion

b) most of the techniques used are thought to activate pain-gating mechanisms and to increase production of brain opiates (endorphins)

3. techniques used in prepared childbirth include

   a) breathing techniques: increase cortical stimulation
      (1) cleansing breath: used before and after contractions
      (2) slow chest breathing: inhale through nose and exhale through mouth; diaphragmatic breathing, used mostly in first stage of labor
      (3) abdominal breathing: abdomen is raised and breath is held during the contraction and exhaled when peak of contraction is passed; used mostly in first stage of labor
      (4) panting: light shallow breathing with mouth open
      (5) pant and blow variations: panting followed by blowing out through pursed lips; helpful during transition and second stage of labor

   b) massage: increases cortical stimulation; effleurage - light stroking by woman of abdomen and thighs

   c) counterpressure may be applied by coach at lower spine or groin

   d) heat or cold may be applied by coach to lower spine

   e) relaxation techniques are used to relax the entire body musculature

   f) maintaining eye contact with coach or using the eyes to focus on a particular object reduces panic and aids in reducing pain stimuli

   g) each stage of labor should use whatever combination of each of the techniques brings the greatest relief of discomfort. Deep chest or abdominal breathing plus relaxation will usually be successful in the first stage of labor. It is during transition period that the woman needs the greatest amount of support and assistance and the greatest amount of controlled activity to reduce discomfort and avoid panic

   h) a variety of positions should be used during labor to increase comfort including walking, standing, side lying pelvic rocking position

   i) when the cervix is fully dilated woman should squat or recline in a semisitting position with knees elevated. After taking a cleansing breath the woman breathes in deeply at start of contraction, holds breath for 5 seconds to fix thoracic and abdominal muscles, and slowly releases the breath as she pushes down with abdominal muscles while relaxing the perineal muscles. She may need to take several breaths during one contraction

III. HYPNOSIS

A. Success depends on client susceptibility to suggestion

B. Requires personnel prepared and trained in hypnotic techniques

IV. NURSING INTERVENTION

A. Assessment of pain
   1. signs of acute pain include
      a) moaning or crying
      b) muscle tension
      c) perspiration
   2. there may be minimal expression of pain even if it is acute in some clients

B. Use a variety of methods to relieve pain
   1. allow the woman to choose the position in which she is most comfortable
      a) in early labor she may be most comfortable ambulating
      b) during the second stage the woman may be most comfortable sitting at a 35-45° angle
      c) lying flat on the back may cause pressure on major blood vessels
   2. explanation to the client what she should expect
      a) knowledge reduces anxiety
   3. teach muscle relaxing exercises
   4. use distraction techniques
      a) as labor intensifies it becomes increasingly difficult to distract client
      b) focusing on object, breathing and relaxation are methods used to distract a client
   5. cutaneous stimulation may encourage relaxation
      a) back rubs
      b) Lamaze type abdominal massage

V. ADVANTAGES

A. Allows for a decreased use of analgesics and anesthesia during labor which decreases probabilities of side effects of these drugs to mother and baby
   1. prepared childbirth does not preclude the judicious use of medication when necessary

B. Intensifies maternal, paternal, child relation by allowing both parents full participation in birth process

C. Knowledge and understanding of childbirth reduces fear, anxiety and pain and makes this experience one of joy

CHAPTER 13

COMPLICATIONS OF LABOR AND DELIVERY

I.  A DIFFICULT LABOR IS CALLED DYSTOCIA

II.  DEVIATIONS IN POWERS AND FORCES

A.  Uterine dysfunction: labor that lasts longer than 24 hours is considered prolonged
1. hypertonic uterine dysfunction formerly known as primary uterine inertia, usually occurs during the latent phase of labor, before active cervical dilation begins
    a) contractions are weak, ineffectual and uncoordinated
    b) the force of the contraction is distorted due to incomplete relaxation of uterine muscles
    c) contractions are painful but do not allow labor to progress
        (1) strength of contraction may be determined by resistance at the abdominal wall to pressure of a finger at the acme of contraction. With a stronger contraction there will not be any indentation of abdominal wall
    d) causes
        (1) muscle weakness and/or nerve defects
        (2) overdistention of uterus (multiple births, hydramnios)
        (3) emotional factors
    e) management
        (1) rest and analgesia
        (2) oxytocics after a period of rest
        (3) enema after rest period

B.  Hypotonic uterine dysfunction formerly known as secondary inertia: occurs during active phase of labor causing ineffectual contractions; labor does not progress
1. contractions are usually short, irregular and infrequent and do not cause much discomfort
2. cause
    a) overdistention of uterus
    b) bladder or bowel distention
    c) weak abdominal muscles
    d) emotional factors
    e) cervical rigidity

f) too early use of analgesia
g) fatigue
h) maternal age and parity
i) pelvic disproportion or fetal malposition
3. management of uterine hypotonic dysfunction
   a) evaluate for disproportion and/or malposition; cesarean section may be indicated if above conditions are implicated
   b) if no abnormality is present oxytocins may be given
   c) amniotomy (artificial rupture of membranes) may be done
   d) IV fluids are usually ordered to prevent dehydration
   e) continuous emotional support and encouragement
   f) provide for patient comfort and rest

C. Dangers to fetus in conditions of uterine dysfunction
1. anoxia
2. injury to brain from constant prolonged pressure on head

D. Danger to mother with uterine dysfunction
1. exhaustion
2. dehydration
3. infection
4. hemorrhage
5. mental strain

E. Pathological retraction ring (Bandl's ring) is an extreme thinning of lower uterine segment with a concomitant thickening of upper segment marked by a ridge (Bandl's ring)
1. danger of rupture of uterus
2. cesarean section is usually indicated

F. Precipitate delivery
1. minimum resistance of soft parts leading to a rapid delivery
2. maternal dangers
   a) lacerations
   b) hemorrhage
   c) infection
3. fetal dangers
   a) anoxia
   b) injuries
   c) infections
4. prevention
   a) those with previous history of rapid labor or high multiparity should be admitted to the hospital early in labor and transferred to the delivery room before full dilation occurs

III. PASSENGER ABNORMALITIES

A. Abnormal positions
  1. occiput posterior
    a) head must rotate in an arc of 135° instead of normal 45° arc
    b) signs
      (1) contractions felt primarily in the back
      (2) almost continuous back pain
      (3) membranes rupture early in labor
      (4) frequent and irregular contractions
      (5) presenting part remains high until late in labor
    c) most posterior presentations will rotate spontaneously
      (1) if spontaneous rotation does not occur persistent posterior may require intervention
      (2) posterior presentation may rotate half way and become a transverse and require intervention
    d) management
      (1) manual rotation may be necessary
      (2) deep mediolateral episiotomy
      (3) forceps may be indicated
      (4) use back massage and positioning to aid in relief of discomfort
    e) excessive molding of fetal head may occur
  2. face-brow
    a) usually caused by any condition which interferes with flexion, i.e., prematurity, short cord, platypelloid pelvis
    b) baby's face or brow is distorted, after delivery, by edema and cyanosis
    c) baby may have hoarseness because of laryngeal edema
    d) danger of maternal hemorrhage following version or high forceps
  3. shoulder (transverse lie)
    a) may rotate spontaneously
    b) podalic version may be done but is dangerous as uterus may rupture
    c) cesarean section usually performed
    d) clinical signs
      (1) abdomen broader than it is long
      (2) head or buttocks may be palpated at pelvic brim
      (3) fundus is empty
    e) prognosis depends upon early diagnosis
      (1) if labor is allowed to continue danger of ruptured uterus or prolapsed cord
      (2) danger of maternal hemorrhage after version or high forceps
  4. prolapsed cord
    a) if presenting part does not fit closely and fill inlet of pelvis danger of prolapse exists
    b) predisposing factors

        (1) breech presentation
        (2) transverse lie
        (3) premature rupture of membranes with floating head
        (4) hydramnios
        (5) pelvic deformity
        (6) multiparity
        (7) premature labor
        (8) long cord
        (9) low lying placenta
    c) prognosis
        (1) labor is not affected
        (2) maternal: no danger
        (3) fetal anoxia
            (a) dependent upon time lapse between prolapse and delivery
            (b) amount of cord compression
    d) management
        (1) prevention
            (a) bed rest after membranes rupture
            (b) membranes should not be ruptured artificially unless head is engaged
        (2) treatment
            (a) if baby is not viable condition is not treated
            (b) if cervix is fully dilated patient is delivered immediately vaginally
            (c) measures for decreasing cord compression and its effects
                1. knee chest position for mother
                2. Trendelenburg position may be preferred
                3. presenting part pushed up vaginally away from cord to prevent cord compression
                4. oxygen by mask to mother
                5. frequent monitoring of fetal heart
                6. patient is told not to bear down
                7. cord is not handled
                    a. no attempt should be made to replace cord
            (d) if cervix is not completely dilated, immediate cesarean section is done
  5. breech presentation (3-4% of pregnancies)
    a) types
        (1) frank breech: buttocks presenting part, with thighs flexed and legs extended (most common)
        (2) complete breech: buttocks presenting part with thighs and knees flexed
        (3) footling: one or both feet present, extension of thighs and knees
        (4) kneeling: knee presents, thighs extended, and knees flexed
    b) etiology
        (1) overdistended uterus
            (a) multiple birth

          (b) hydramnios
          (c) hydrocephalus
          (d) large baby
          (e) pelvic abnormality which interferes with the en-
              largement of the head
       (2) premature baby
       (3) placenta previa
     c) clinical manifestations
       (1) head is at fundus
       (2) fetal heart at or above umbilicus
       (3) engagement usually does not occur
       (4) membranes rupture early
       (5) meconium stained amniotic fluid
     d) prognosis
       (1) maternal: no significantly greater mortality
          (a) may have prolonged labor
          (b) if delivery is spontaneous no increase in trauma
             to perineal area
          (c) increased incidence of forceps delivery which
             may cause trauma to perineal area
       (2) baby: fetal loss three times higher than in vertex
          presentation
          (a) asphyxia
          (b) brain injury due to rapid delivery of head
          (c) skeletal injury
          (d) premature separation of placenta
     e) management of breech
       (1) reduce incidence of complications by x-ray pelvim-
          etry or sonogram
       (2) constant monitoring of FHR and maternal status
       (3) cesarean section performed if (Reeder, et al., 1980)
          (a) fetus is larger than 8.5 lbs
          (b) there is fetopelvic disproportion
          (c) labor does not progress
          (d) fetal distress occurs

B.    Fetal abnormalities may lead to necessity for cesarean sec-
     tion
     1. hydrocephalus: enlargement of the cranium due to exces-
       sive accumulation of CSF
     2. anencephaly: abnormally small cranium due to the absence
       of cranial bones and/or portions of the brain
     3. oversized baby
     4. postmaturity (bones do not mold easily)
     5. edema of fetus (hydrops fetalis)
     6. short umbilical cord
       a) less than 20 inches is abnormal
       b) may be twisted rather than short
       c) fetus cannot descend
       d) may cause anoxia

C.  Multiple pregnancy may cause
    1. overdistention of uterus
    2. postpartal hemorrhage
    3. premature births to have an increased incidence
    4. general anesthesia to be contraindicated

IV.  PLACENTAL ABNORMALITIES

A.  Retained placenta
    1. placenta separates but is held by contracted cervix
    2. management
       a) manual removal

B.  Adherent placenta
    1. placenta doesn't separate, needs manual separation and
       removal

C.  Placenta accreta (extremely rare)
    1. villi of placenta invade muscles of uterus
    2. no blood loss unless manual removal is attempted
    3. persistent attempt at removal may lead to
       a) hemorrhage
       b) perforation or rupture of uterus
       c) shock
    4. management
       a) conservative
          (1) left alone to absorb
          (2) antibiotic therapy
          (3) oxytocin administered
       b) radical
          (1) if bleeding is uncontrollable, hysterectomy is per-
              formed

V.  ABNORMALITIES OF PASSAGE

A.  Uterus
    1. developmental
       a) double uterus (bicornate): full term pregnancy ex-
          tremely rare with this condition
    2. displacement
       a) ventrofixation: cervix is displaced in region of sacral
          promontory
          (1) if cervix cannot be repositioned, cesarean section
              is necessary
    3. tumors (fibroids and neoplasms)
       a) block pelvis
       b) cause malpresentations
       c) do not allow for adequate contractions
       d) may necessitate cesarean section

B.  Cervix
    1. may be rigid or resistant due to

a) scar tissue
b) chronic inflammation
c) rigid tissue (elderly primipara over 35)
d) if dilation does not progress cesarean section may be necessary

C. Vagina
1. congenital malformations
2. acquired obstruction
a) cystocele and rectocele
3. may impede delivery

D. Vulva
1. edema
a) irritation from antiseptics
b) may cause extreme discomfort to patient

E. Bony pelvis
1. may be contracted or deformed
2. clinical manifestations depend on
a) degree of contraction
b) size of fetus
3. management
a) trial labor
b) cesarean section if indicated

VI. OPERATIVE OBSTETRICS

A. Cesarean section: child is delivered through an incision in the abdominal and uterine walls
1. incidence of cesarean sections increasing because of
a) increased use of fetal monitoring diagnoses fetal distress more accurately
b) changing philosophy of management of labor
(1) minimize fetal trauma in breech presentation
(2) prolonged labor will increase stress to mother and fetus
(3) prevent sepsis when there is premature rupture of membranes
(4) pregnancies in which there is an unfavorable uterine environment will be terminated because of the advances in newborn intensive care
(5) advances in anesthesia, blood replacement and antibiotics makes cesarean section delivery method of choice in some complications of pregnancy
(6) controversy surrounds the increased incidence and efforts to control overuse are currently being investigated
c) indications
(1) any condition which precludes vaginal delivery
(2) repeat sections are left to the discretion of the physician

        (a) vaginal delivery may be considered after a previous cesarean delivery
- (3) placenta previa
- (4) premature separation of placenta
- (5) toxemia
- (6) diabetes
- (7) fetal distress

2. management
   a) preoperative care
     (1) insertion of Foley catheter to prevent accidental injury to bladder
     (2) abdominal and pubic prep
     (3) preoperative medication as ordered
        (a) atropine is usually ordered
        (b) narcotic drugs are avoided because they are CNS depressants
     (4) preparation of back because spinal anesthesia is anesthesia best suited to procedure
     (5) type and x-match of blood
     (6) routine lab studies
     (7) general physical exam
     (8) consent form signed
     (9) explanation of rationale for section and what to expect during the procedure to the client and her family
    (10) continued observation of FHR and maternal vital signs
   b) immediate postoperative care
     (1) maintain airway if general anesthesia is used
     (2) monitor vital signs
     (3) monitor intake and output
        (a) check patency of Foley catheter
        (b) check IVs for rate or infiltration
     (4) relief of pain
     (5) hygienic care
     (6) maintain body alignment if spinal anesthesia is used
     (7) encourage deep breathing
     (8) if spinal anesthesia is used head should remain flat for 8-12 hours
     (9) observation for hemorrhage and shock
    (10) massage of fundus is contraindicated
    (11) oxytocics administered as ordered

3. psychosocial impact of cesarean section
   a) may be relieved that labor is over, but may feel failure or defeat
   b) may undergo a grieving process
     (1) loss of vaginal delivery
     (2) loss of active participation in labor process
   c) increased anxiety about their welfare and that of their child
   d) increase in fatigue and pain

e) may need more time to meet her own dependency needs
f) support of spouse and significant others facilitates recovery
g) may have influence on future childbearing

B. Forceps
  1. indications
    a) prolonged labor, fetal or maternal condition weakened
    b) prolapsed cord
    c) fetal distress
  2. criteria
    a) no cephalopelvic disproportion
    b) cervix should be completely dilated
    c) membranes must be ruptured
    d) fetal head must be engaged
    e) bladder must be emptied
    f) if any of these conditions are not met, forceps should
       not be used
  3. types of forceps
    a) outlet or low forceps
      (1) head is on the pelvic floor and is crowning
        (a) some of the benefits are believed to be
          1. more controlled delivery
          2. less exposure of head to pressure against the
             perineum
          3. minimization of trauma to maternal tissues
    b) mid-forceps
      (1) head is engaged
      (2) some manipulation necessary
        (a) usually rotation of head
      (3) dangers associated with forceps delivery depend upon
        (a) position and level of presenting part
        (b) skill of the obstetrician
    c) high-forceps: head not engaged
      (1) this procedure is no longer justified, cesarean sec-
          tion is safer

C. Vacuum extraction: more popular in Europe
  1. occasionally used in place of forceps
  2. a metal cup (varying sizes) applied to fetal head and air is
     withdrawn by pump to create a vacuum
  3. vacuum is built up slowly
  4. traction exerted by a steady pull on cup
  5. depending on the duration and extent of pulling, swelling of
     head will develop with some bruising

D. Episiotomy
  1. indications
    a) to prevent perineal lacerations
  2. types
    a) midline
    b) right or left mediolateral

      3. the routine use of episiotomy to prevent laceration has been questioned since in many cases careful management of delivery can prevent lacerations

VII. INDUCTION AND AUGMENTATION OF LABOR

A. Use of agent to bring about labor or use agent to increase the speed and intensity of labor

B. Indications
    1. postmaturity
    2. maternal diabetes or preeclampsia
    3. uterine inertia
    4. ruptured membranes for more than 24 hours
    5. management of incomplete, inevitable or missed abortion

C. Contraindications
    1. high parity
    2. previous cesarean section
    3. multiple births
    4. first baby
    5. cephalopelvic disproportion
    6. abnormal presentation
    7. overdistention of uterus
    8. fetal distress
    9. unfavorable fetal presentation
  10. hypersensitivity to drug

D. Types of induction
    1. amniotomy: allows presenting part to become a more effective dilating wedge
    2. use of amniotomy as a means of induction is being seriously reconsidered
       a) if there is a long period of time elapsed between amniotomy and delivery, there is danger of infection
       b) there is a danger that labor will not follow rupture of membranes
    3. management of amniotomy
       a) prepare client for vaginal examination
       b) maintain sterile technique
       c) immediately after procedure check
          (1) amniotic fluid for meconium
          (2) fetal heart

E. Drugs used for induction
    1. synthetic preparations of oxytocic
       a) various trade names include Pitocin and Syntocinon
       b) given by IV drip
          (1) usual dose is 5–10 U diluted in 1000 cc of appropriate IV fluid
             (a) when 1 IU of oxytocin is added to 1000 ml of IV fluid each ml contains 1 mU of oxytocin. 1 IU = 1000 milliunits (mU)

      (2) IV bottle should be clearly labeled with
         (a) name of drug
         (b) amount of drug
         (c) time drug added
   c) piggyback set-up should be used so that oxytocic administration can be immediately halted and there is an open vein for emergency
      (1) the IV should be administered very slowly and response closely monitored
      (2) any contractions lasting more than one minute or occurring less than 2 minutes apart necessitates immediate adjustment of medication administration
      (3) careful observation of patient reaction to drug fetal heart rate and vital signs
      (4) constant physician supervision of drug administration is necessary
      (5) IV discontinued immediately if any untoward signs occur
         (a) contraction lasting over 90 seconds
         (b) abnormalities in FH
   d) danger of severe and prolonged contraction exists
      (1) may cause uterine tetany (tetanic contraction - no relaxation)
         (a) rupture of uterus
         (b) premature placental separation
         (c) fetal hypoxia
   e) observation of mother's pulse, blood pressure, as well as monitoring of contractions and fetal heart rate every 15 minutes is important
2. a new type of drug for inducing labor is called prostaglandins
   a) naturally occurring substances in the human body about which little is now known
   b) mode of action is not known but prostaglandins E1, E2, and F2a have been shown to stimulate uterine activity at term
   c) effect on uterine activity by prostaglandins is slower than Pitocin but persists for 10 to 30 minutes after drug is discontinued
   d) use of this drug is experimental at this time
   e) has not been approved by the FDA for routine use in labor
3. oxytocin challenge test (OCT): assesses the ability of the fetus to withstand labor
   a) labor stimulated by dilute concentration of oxytocic
   b) FHR and uterine contractions measured to see response
      (1) negative test: no periodic late decelerations
      (2) positive test: deceleration patterns indicate that fetal status is compromised by mild contractions
         (a) fetus may not be able to withstand labor
   c) OCT may be administered weekly or biweekly from about

the thirty-fourth week of gestation in high risk pregnancies
  d) woman near term may go into spontaneous labor
  e) nursing intervention
    (1) careful monitoring
    (2) emotional and physical support as with a patient in
        labor

F.  Preterm labor (Pritchard and MacDonald, 1980)
  1. occurs between the twentieth and thirty-fourth week of ges-
     tation
  2. results in effacement and dilation
  3. causes
    a) spontaneous rupture of membranes
    b) cervical incompetency
    c) uterine anomalies
    d) hydramnios
    e) multiple birth
    f) fetal anomaly
    g) placenta abruptio or previa
    h) fetal death
    i) previous preterm delivery or late abortion
    j) systemic disease in the mother
  4. management
    a) bedrest
    b) IV ethanol
      (1) suppresses oxytocin and vasopressin from maternal
          posterior pituitary
      (2) crosses the placenta
        (a) fetal blood level of alcohol equals those of the
            mother within 2 hours
      (3) side effects include
        (a) intoxication of mother
        (b) nausea, vomiting
        (c) headache
        (d) restlessness
        (e) hypoglycemia and lactic acidemia
        (f) may cause respiratory distress in newborn if la-
            bor is not arrested
      (4) contraindicated
        (a) liver disease
        (b) reformed alcoholics
        (c) must be used with extreme caution in women with
            epilepsy and diabetes
    c) magnesium sulfate
      (1) inhibits smooth muscle contractability
      (2) crosses the placenta
        (a) concentration in fetal plasma rapidly reaches
            that of the mother
      (3) side effects include
        (a) warmth, flushing

        (b) headache
        (c) pulmonary edema
        (d) perspiration
        (e) respiratory depression
        (f) neonatal depression
   d) ritrodrine (PDR, 1981)
     (1) beta-adrenergic stimulant
     (2) inhibits smooth muscle contractibility
     (3) side effects include
        (a) nervousness, restlessness, anxiety
        (b) chest pain, hypotension
        (c) hyperventilations
        (d) pulmonary edema
        (e) increase in FHR
        (f) fetal hypocalcemia
        (g) fetal hypoglycemia
     (4) contraindication
        (a) maternal hemorrhage
        (b) eclampsia and severe preeclampsia
        (c) chorioamnionitis
        (d) intrauterine fetal death
        (e) maternal cardiac disease, pulmonary hyperten-
           sion, hyperthyroidism and uncontrolled diabetes
        (f) sensitivity to drug
        (g) maternal conditions that would be adversely af-
           fected
   e) prostaglandins inhibitors
     (1) may prevent synthesis of prostaglandin or block ac-
        tion on target cells
     (2) affects all organ systems
     (3) side-effects
        (a) nausea, vertigo, allergic reactions
        (b) gastrointestinal complications
        (c) neonatal pulmonary hypotension
        (d) cardiovascular changes in fetus
           1. "extensive investigation in humans of the use
             of prostaglandin synthesis inhibitors to try to
             inhibit preterm labor has been discouraged
             following recognition that such agents may ad-
             versely affect the fetus" (Pritchard and Mac-
             Donald, 1980)
5. nursing intervention
   a) education of the woman regarding
     (1) factors that lead to preterm labor
     (2) signs and symptoms of preterm labor
   b) if the woman is hospitalized (Herron and Dulock, unpub-
     lished)
     (1) put the woman on bedrest on her left side in Trendel-
        enburg position
        (a) left side position maximizes uterine blood flow
        (b) Trendelenburg may alleviate cervical pressure

          (2) assess the woman for, include notation of time of onset, duration and severity
            (a) backache
            (b) cramping
            (c) uterine contractions
            (d) vaginal discharge
          (3) if on ritodrine, monitor for pulmonary edema and respiratory distress syndrome, also avoid overhydration
         (4) provide emotional support and give realistic reassurance

## VIII. ACCIDENTS AND INJURIES IN LABOR AND DELIVERY

A. Lacerations
   1. cervical: sulcus tear extends to cervix from perineum
     a) increased possibility of hemorrhage if not adequately repaired
     b) surgical repair and vaginal packing is used
   2. perineal
     a) first degree: perineal skin, fourchette and mucous membrane
     b) second degree: muscles of perineal body
     c) third degree: includes rectal sphincter
     d) surgical repair at time of delivery
     e) may be prevented by judicious use of episiotomy and careful, slow delivery of the head

B. Rupture of uterus
   1. causes
     a) contracted pelvis
     b) Bandl's ring
     c) previous cesarean section
     d) improper use of instruments
     e) improper use of oxytocin
   2. symptoms of impending rupture
     a) continuous contractions
     b) restlessness
     c) bladder appears full but patient cannot void - not relieved by catheterization
     d) uterus tender
   3. symptoms of acute rupture
     a) sharp tearing pain in lower abdomen (feeling of something tearing)
     b) pain ceases
     c) hemorrhage and shock quickly follow
   4. should not be allowed to occur; careful observation can prevent rupture
   5. if it occurs hysterectomy may be done

C. Inversion of uterus (turned inside out)
   1. etiology

a) usually trauma, i.e., pulling on cord or fundal pressure
b) may be spontaneous
2. dangers
   a) shock
   b) hemorrhage
   c) infection
   d) high mortality rate
3. management
   a) replacement of uterus
   b) blood replacement

D. Sudden death in labor
   1. causes
      a) anesthesia
      b) aspiration
      c) amniotic fluid embolism
      d) transfusion reaction
      e) C.V.A.

IX. NURSING CARE DURING COMPLICATIONS OF LABOR AND DELIVERY

A. Assessment
   1. directed toward detecting early signs and symptoms of possible and potential problems
      a) contractions
         (1) frequency
         (2) duration
         (3) intensity
      b) vaginal discharge
         (1) color
         (2) amount
         (3) character
      c) vital signs
      d) stress and anxiety level
      e) abdominal contour
      f) fetal heart rate
      g) fatigue and exhaustion
      h) abnormal pain

B. Intervention
   1. intervention is based on an understanding and interpretation of the assessment
   2. immediate reporting of any deviation from normal
   3. explanation of status to the client and her family
   4. realistic reassurance as to outcome of labor and delivery
   5. explanation of procedures
   6. encouragement as to progress
   7. provide an atmosphere where client and family can freely verbalize their fears and concerns

## STUDY QUESTIONS

1. The patient has been pregnant five times. She had one spontaneous abortion, one stillborn full term and two living children. When she is admitted to the hospital labor her record reads Grav _____ Para _____
2. Examination of the patient reveals that there is a vertex presentation, in the R.O.P. position, zero station, cervix thinning and 5 cm dilated. What does this mean?
3. Why is the patient NPO in labor?
4. Why is it essential to prevent bladder distention during labor?
5. What is the normal fetal heart range?
6. What should be checked immediately following amniotomy?
7. How should uterine contractions be timed?
8. During the first stage of labor, what symptoms should be immediately reported to physician?
9. When is induction of labor contraindicated?
10. What special precautions must be taken during an induction?
11. During what stage of labor should bearing down be encouraged?
12. Which method of anesthesia is least harmful to the infant?
13. What are the advantages of natural childbirth? The disadvantages?
14. What are some factors that cause uterine dystocia?
15. What symptoms indicate that uterine rupture is imminent?
16. What five physiological functions are evaluated in the Apgar score?
17. What are the signs of fetal distress?
18. What observations are essential during the fourth stage of labor?
19. If the uterus relaxes after delivery, what nursing action should be taken?

## BIBLIOGRAPHY

Allen, S.: Nurse Attendance During Labor, American Journal of Nursing, July, 1964.

Bender, A.: A Test of the Effect of Nursing Support on Mothers in Labor, A.N.A. Regional Clinical Conference, 1967.

Case, Lynda, L.: Ultrasound Monitoring of Mother and Fetus, American Journal of Nursing, April, 1972.

Clark, Ann, Affonso, Dyanne: Childbearing: A Nursing Perspective. F.A. Davis Co., Phila., 1979.

Cohen, S.N.: Drugs that Depress the Newborn Infant, Pediatric Clinics of North America, Volume 17, November, 1970.

Greiss, Frank: Obstetric Analgesia and Anesthesia, American Journal of Nursing, January, 1971.

Jenson, M., Benson, R., and Bobak, I.: Maternity Care - The Nurse and the Family, St. Louis, The C.V. Mosby Company, 1977.

Johnson, Grace: Oxytocics for the Induction of Labor, N.Y., March of Dimes, 1981.

Kopp, L.: Ordeal or Ideal - The Second Stage of Labor, American Journal of Nursing, June, 1971.

Laros, R., Work, B., Witting, W.: Prostaglandins, American Journal of Nursing, June, 1973.

Lasater, Carol: Electronic Monitoring of Mother and Fetus, American Journal of Nursing, April, 1972.

Leboyer, Frederick: Birth Without Violence, Alfred A. Knopf, N.Y., 1975.

Liu, Yuen Chou: Effects of an Upright Position During Labor, American Journal of Nursing, December, 1974.

Lum, B., Batzel, R., and Barnett, E.: Reappraising Newborn Eye Care, American Journal of Nursing, September, 1980, pp. 1602-1603.

Oxorn, H. and Foote, W.: Human Labor and Birth, Appleton-Century-Crofts, N.Y., 1964.

Physicians Desk Reference (PDR) (35th Ed.): Oradel, N.J., Medical Economics Co., 1981.

Pilon, Robert: Anesthesia for Uncomplicated Obstetric Delivery, American Family Physician, January, 1974.

Pohodich, Jane: Selected Drugs used During Labor and Delivery: Effects on the Fetus and Neonate, N.Y. March of Dimes, 1980.

Pritchard, J. and MacDonald, P.: Williams Obstetrics, 16th Ed., N.Y., Appleton-Century-Crofts, 1980.

Reeder, S., Mastroianni, L., Martin, L., Fitzpatrick, E., Maternity Nursing, J.B. Lippincott Company, Phila., 1980.

Rich, O.: Hospital Routines as Rites of Passage in Developing Maternal Identity, Nursing Clinics of North American, Vol. 4, 1969.

Rising, Sharon: The Fourth Stage of Labor: Family Integration. American Journal of Nursing, May, 1974.

Russin, A., O'Gureck, J., Roux, J.: Electronic Monitoring of the Fetus, American Journal of Nursing, July, 1974.

Sasmor, J., et al.: The Childbirth Team During Labor, American Journal of Nursing, March, 1973.

Shainess, Natalie: The Psychologic Experience of Labor, N.Y. State Journal of Medicine, October, 1963.

Smith, B., et al.: The Transition Phase of Labor, American Journal of Nursing, March, 1973.

CHAPTER 14

ANATOMY AND PHYSIOLOGY OF THE PUERPERIUM

I.  DEFINITION OF PUERPERIUM - 6-12 week period from the end of labor to the complete involution of uterus and healing of pelvic structures

II. PHYSIOLOGICAL AND ANATOMICAL CHANGES

A.  Uterus
    1. size and position after delivery
       a) fundus hard, globular and contracted, usually felt at umbilicus if bladder not distended
       b) usual weight 1000 g
    2. after delivery the uterus descends into pelvic cavity approximately one centimeter a day.  By the tenth day, fundus usually cannot be palpated
    3. at the end of puerperium weight of uterus is 40-60 g
    4. process of involution is accomplished by
       a) autolysis of protein of uterine lining.  Waste products are excreted in urine causing albuminuria
       b) two layers of decidua are involved in involution
          (1) one is cast off as lochia
          (2) underlying layer becomes endometrial lining
              (a) entire endometrium restored by third week
       c) placental site: completely regenerated within 6 weeks
       d) large uterine blood vessels become smaller
       e) well contracted uterus clamps down on maternal blood vessels and controls hemorrhage
       f) uterus is a very tactile organ immediately after delivery and responds to massage by contracting
       g) involution occurs more rapidly in primipara or breast feeding mother because of increased muscle tone in primipara and release of oxytocin during breast feeding
       h) factors delaying involution
          (1) multiparity
          (2) conditions causing overdistention of uterus
              (a) hydramnios
              (b) large-sized baby
          (3) infection
          (4) retained placenta or membranes
          (5) hormonal deficiencies

171

i) subinvolution occurs when uterus fails to return to normal size

B.  Cervix
1. immediately after delivery cervix is soft, flabby and partly open
2. after 1 week muscle begins to regenerate and finger cannot be introduced
3. small lacerations may heal spontaneously or need cauterization
4. external os remains somewhat wider than the nonparous woman

C.  Lochia: contains blood from placental site, decidua, cervical secretions, epithelial cells and bacteria
1. Lochia rubra: 1-4 days; bright red
    a) if persists longer than 2 weeks, may indicate retained placenta or membranes
2. Lochia serosa: 4-10 days; pinkish brown in color
3. Lochia alba: 10-14 day; whitish discharge due to increase in leucocytes
4. should not be excessive, scant (during rubra) or foul smelling
5. blood clots may be passed immediately after delivery

D.  Perineum
1. vaginal distention decreases, but muscle tone never returns to preparous state
2. lacerations, tears, sutures, swellings gradually heal

E.  Abdominal wall
1. soft and flabby for some time
2. striae fade to silvery white, but always remain
3. diastasis of the recti muscle (separation of abdominal muscle) may occur due to loss of muscle tone

F.  Urinary tract
1. ureteral dilation disappears in two weeks
2. increased output (diuresis) second to fifth day due to excretion of extracellular fluid
3. urine may contain increased amounts of acetone, (CHO breakdown) nitrogen, and albumin (protein autolysis of uterus), and lactose from production of mammary glands
4. urethera and ureters become slightly dilated and edematous

G.  Breasts
1. soft immediately after delivery
2. high levels of estrogen and progesterone secreted by placenta inhibit anterior pituitary secretion
3. after delivery of placenta inhibition is removed and lactogenic hormone (prolactin) is secreted which stimulates

production of milk

a) synthetic estrogen and androgens given intramuscularly immediately after delivery suppress lactogenic hormones in patients who do not wish to breast feed

4. 2 days postpartum, engorgement of breasts may occur

a) caused by venous and lymphatic secretion stasis
b) various degrees of engorgement occur
c) in most severe type, breasts are swollen, hard, red, and painful

H. Blood

1. decrease in volume following blood loss in delivery
2. hemodilution of blood (hydremia) is decreased in first week postpartum through excretion by kidneys and from skin
3. moderate anemia may occur due to blood loss
4. leukocytosis occurs during labor and immediately afterwards
5. fibrinogen levels are elevated
6. immediately after delivery, pulse rate slows

I. Weight loss

1. usually 10-12 pounds immediately after delivery, 13 pounds more are gradually lost after the initial loss
2. loss of weight due to

a) delivery of baby and placenta
b) hydremia reduction
c) excretion of retained fluid
d) uterine involution

3. although back to normal weight, patient may appear obese because of poor abdominal muscle tone

J. Skin

1. mask of pregnancy gradually fades
2. linea nigra fades but never disappears
3. striae fades but remains silvery white
4. primary areola may never resume original color
5. secondary areola fades in 3 months

K. Hormonal

1. nonlactating woman

a) ovulation within 3-6 weeks
b) menstruation within 5-8 weeks

2. lactating woman

a) return of menstrual cycle varies; may be delayed until weaning
b) because of variation, breast feeding is not a reliable form of contraception

# CHAPTER 15

## PSYCHOLOGY OF THE PUERPERIUM

I. FACTORS INFLUENCING ADJUSTMENT TO NEW ROLE

A. Change in metabolism
   1. tremendous drop in hormonal levels of estrogen and pro-
      gesterone

B. New sense of responsibility may be influenced by
   1. maturity of new parents
   2. fear of failure to measure up to ideal parent role
   3. lack of knowledge of newborn
   4. financial worries
   5. marital relationships

C. Attention diverted from mother to baby

D. Development of maternal instinct and bonding may be delayed
   1. analgesia and anesthesia which precludes experiencing the
      birth process, and immediate separation of mother and
      child may be a factor in this delay

E. In out-of-wedlock mother guilt, shame, and feelings of hos-
   tility toward child may be present and may have an influence
   on the maternal-child relationship

III. STAGES IN ADJUSTMENT TO NEW ROLE

A. Immediately after delivery there is a need for sleep which if
   interrupted, causes patient to experience sleep hunger
   1. after natural childbirth, patient may be so exhilarated, she
      may not be aware of her own exhaustion

B. Classification of phase of puerperal restoration according to
   Reva Rubin (1961)
   1. taking-in phase
      a) lasts 2-3 days
      b) mother passive and dependent
      c) expresses own needs rather than baby's
         (1) in order for mother to meet baby's needs, her own
             needs must be met

174

(2) needs physical care and attention to her emotional needs

d) verbalizes reactions to delivery so that experience can be integrated

e) symbiotic relationship ends and child should begin to be recognized as an individual

2. taking-hold phase
   a) third to tenth day
   b) the mother strives for independence and autonomy - she wants to care for herself and her child
   c) initiates action
   d) strong anxiety element
      (1) unsure of mothering role
      (2) unsure of ability to physically care for child
   e) develop maternal responsibilities and feelings
   f) mother may experience rapid and frequent mood swings
      (1) she may have ambivalent feelings about the baby
   g) curious and interested in care of baby
   h) stage of maximum readiness for new learning

3. letting-go phase
   a) from 2 week postdelivery to several months
   b) infant is perceived as on individual separate from the mother
   c) both parents adjust to their new parental role
   d) ambivalent feelings about parenthood and about their readiness for their new role will be present
   e) parents attempt to adjust to changes in their lifestyle that parenting brings

C. Establishment of new role
   1. the birth of a baby may be viewed as a developmental crisis
      a) roles are reassigned
      b) new responsibilities added
      c) values reoriented
      d) needs are met in new ways
   2. LeMaster's study revealed that new parents have not been adequately prepared for new role and may have difficulties in adjustment (LeMasters, 1965)
      a) mother's relationship to husband changes
      b) father may feel isolation, economic pressure, dissatisfaction with paternal role
      c) mother may feel fatigued, may have decrease in satisfaction due to confinement in home, loss of social contacts, burden of additional household duties and guilt about not being a "better mother"

D. Maternal-child interaction
   1. immediately after delivery the mother may not have grasped the reality of the birth

2. the mother will react to the infant according to her perceptions of its needs. This perception will be based on the child's
    a) sex
    b) activity level
    c) appearance
    d) size
3. the first interaction between mother and infant is one of exploration and examination
    a) a primipara will usually explore with hand and fingers
    b) a multipara will usually enfold the infant using her arms as extensions of her body
4. initial behavior is usually concerned with ability to function in mothering role
    a) a primipara in her first contact may show signs of tension
       (1) flushed face
       (2) excessive perspiration
       (3) body rigid
       (4) may be anxious for baby to be taken away
5. maternal cues which indicate acceptance and claiming of infant as her own
    a) assigns cultural values regarding sex
    b) identifies resemblance of baby to family members
    c) calls baby by name
    d) touching and fondling child
    e) assumes en face position with baby

E.   Paternal-child interaction
     1. may exhibit fear and anxiety about handling baby
     2. may show positive reactions similar to mother

III.  POSTPARTAL BLUES

A.   Incidence may be decreasing due to
     1. better obstetrical care
     2. better preparation for new role
     3. allowing verbalization of feelings

B.   Timing and severity of symptoms vary with the individual
     1. usually comes on within 2 weeks of childbirth and ends within 3 months

C.   Manifestations
     1. loss of energy
     2. crying
     3. anxiety, fear, and confusion
     4. insomnia (may indicate more serious emotional upset)
     5. concerned about her body
     6. misinterpretation of actions and words of others, primarily her husband

    7. extreme control
        a) insists everything is okay

D.  Theories of etiology
    1. stress of labor and birth
    2. hormonal changes
        a) placental secretion ceases
        b) lactation begins
        c) new research shows an association between postpartal
           blues and high levels of estrogen, low levels of proges-
           terone and abnormal levels of other hormones postpar-
           tally
    3. immaturity
    4. family, social and economic problems
    5. need for rest ignored
        a) overstimulation leads to lack of sleep and exhaustion
           which may bring about feelings of depression

E.  Mother may verbalize
    1. a sensation of feeling unprotected
    2. a feeling of emptiness
        a) removal of baby may be compared to amputation

CHAPTER 16

NURSING CARE DURING PUERPERIUM

I.    NURSING GOALS

A.    The major goals of nursing during the puerperium are
      1. assist in maternal restoration of physiological and psycho-
         logical status
      2. assist parents in adjusting to and accepting new roles
      3. assist in parent-child bonding so that an adequate parent-
         child relationship can be formed

II.   ASSESSMENT AND INTERVENTION

A.    Assessment and intervention are based on the physiological
      and psychological changes occurring during the puerperium

B.    Assessment and intervention for restoration of physiological
      status
      1. uterine involution
         a) fundus is checked daily for position and tone
            (1) mother should be instructed to relax abdominal mus-
                cles during palpation of the fundus to reduce possi-
                ble discomfort during the procedure
            (2) palpate the uterus by placing the side of one hand on
                top of and cupped slightly behind the top of the fun-
                dus, and placing the other hand on the bottom of the
                uterus suprapubically with very slight pressure to
                provide support
            (3) before palpating the fundus observe to see if there is
                a full bladder (bladder bulge over the symphysis pu-
                bis). Bladder should be emptied before palpation or
                massage of fundus
            (4) when assessing fundal tone and position consider the
                influence of infant size, length of labor, hydramnios
                and multiple births. Fundus of a multipara will usu-
                ally be larger and higher than a primipara
            (5) first day p.p. fundus should be at or below the um-
                bilicus at midline of abdomen
            (6) fundus continues to descend each day until it can no
                longer be palpated (usually by the tenth day)
                (a) involution will be slower in multiparas

178

      (7) fundus should remain firm and well contracted at all times

      (8) bladder distention will inhibit involution and may push fundus to the side of the abdomen

   b) check color, amount and odor of lochia

      (1) should proceed from bright red to white discharge

   c) after-pains primarily in multiparas or may occur in primiparas if blood clots form

      (1) decreased uterine muscle tone makes it difficult to maintain a state of tonic contraction. When uterus relaxes slightly at intervals, strong contractions occur to return uterus to well contracted state

      (2) usually subsides within 48 hours

      (3) the uterus contracts when the mother sees or hears her infant and after oxytocic drugs are administered

2. intervention

   a) if relaxation occurs, massage is done to return uterus to well contracted state

      (1) massage should be gentle and any blood clots expressed

         (a) to express blood clots, apply pressure with one hand to fundus with equal pressure applied to bottom of uterus above symphysis pubis and apply pressure for a few seconds with periods of rest between intervals until blood clot has been expressed

         (b) if fundus is baggy, massage gently with a circular motion on top and slightly in back of top of uterus until fundus contracts firmly. Always support bottom of uterus with one hand during massage

      (2) overstimulation of uterus through massage should be avoided as it may lead to muscle fatigue and relaxation of the uterus

      (3) if massage is ineffective, physician should be notified

   b) oxytocics are given to assist involution

   c) breast feeding assists involution

   d) medication to relieve pain is given when necessary for after-pains

      (1) abdominal breathing exercises may be beneficial

      (2) explanation of causes of pain and reassurance as to transient nature of pain is helpful

   e) if involution fails to proceed normally, the physician should be notified

   f) bladder distention should be avoided

3. postpartum chill

   a) may occur immediately after delivery

   b) not followed by fever

   c) theories of etiology

      (1) nervous reaction combined with exhaustion following birth

- (2) disequilibrium between internal and external temperatures caused by
  - (a) perspiration during labor
  - (b) loss of body fluids
  - (c) change of intraabdominal pressure
- d) nursing intervention
  - (1) keep patient warm
  - (2) reassure
4. sleep
  - a) immediately postpartum, the new mother needs deep, long, uninterrupted sleep
    - (1) patient should be placed in a quiet, darkened room
    - (2) patient should be disturbed as little as possible
  - b) subsequent sleep and rest patterns should be monitored through the assessment of
    - (1) mother's statements
    - (2) nurses' observations
  - c) hinderances to sleep
    - (1) perineal soreness
    - (2) hemorrhoids
    - (3) after-pains
    - (4) anxiety
  - d) interventions
    - (1) relieve any discomforts
    - (2) allow mother to verbalize anxieties
    - (3) reduce environmental noise during night
    - (4) plan nursing care to allow for daytime rest period and early morning sleep
    - (5) analgesia and sedatives may be provided when other comfort measures fail
5. perineal healing
  - a) etiology of trauma
    - (1) lacerations
    - (2) suturing
    - (3) hemorrhoids
    - (4) hematomas
  - b) assessment of the perineal area is done daily by visual inspection. Check for
    - (1) degree of inflammation and signs of infection
    - (2) swelling
    - (3) discoloration
    - (4) discharge around area of trauma
    - (5) abnormal odors
    - (6) patients subjective feelings of discomfort should be considered
    - (7) healing process
  - c) intervention
    - (1) sitz bath (only with physician's orders)
    - (2) infrared lamp (only with physician's orders)
    - (3) if there is a hematoma, ice pack offers some relief; if applied early may prevent hematoma

(4) suppositories to relieve discomforts of hemorrhoids (only with physician's orders)
(5) rubber ring to relieve pressure on perineal area
(6) exercise to increase blood circulation to perineal area and increase muscle tone
    (a) Kegels contractions: contract and relax muscles alternately as if starting and stopping urinary flow can be done in any position and should be repeated frequently
(7) personal hygiene
    (a) mother is usually bathed and given perineal care soon after delivery
    (b) perineal care is done by nurse and is taught to patient when she is capable of assuming responsibility
        1. purpose is to prevent infection, cleanse area, and provide soothing warmth
        2. cleansing during perineal care should be based on principles of asepsis

6. reestablishment of bladder and bowel function
  a) assessment of bladder function
    (1) distended bladder is recognized by bulge under uterus and displacement of uterus upward and laterally
    (2) measure first voiding to rule out retention with overflow (over 100 cc)
    (3) continuous observation of intake and output
    (4) check for signs of infection
        (a) pain or burning on voiding
    (5) check concentration of urinary output by assessing color, quantity and odor
  b) intervention
    (1) inability to void is a common problem
        (a) etiology
            1. long labor and/or traumatic delivery
            2. swelling of perineal area around urethra
            3. poor bladder tone due to pressure
            4. reflex spasm of bladder sphincter due to pain
            5. fatigue
            6. diminished sensitivity due to drugs and anesthesia
            7. emotional factors (fear of letting go)
    (2) encourage patient to void by usual methods
    (3) maintain adequate fluid intake
    (4) catheterization if indicated as ordered
        (a) with extreme bladder distention (over 1000 cc) do not completely empty bladder to prevent possibility of shock
    (5) record amount of first voiding
  c) assessment of bowel function
    (1) may be constipated

          (a) caused by decreased intra-abdominal pressure and relaxation of abdominal muscles

          (b) mother may be afraid to have bowel movement because of

            1. pain from soreness of perineal area

            2. fear of rupturing sutures

   d) intervention

     (1) encourage mother to take the time to have first bowel movement

     (2) support perineal area with pad while bearing down

     (3) encourage fluid and high fiber intake

     (4) use cathartics and enemas as necessary

7. breasts

   a) assessment

     (1) determine whether mother will breast feed

     (2) engorgement

     (3) nipple inversion or cracking

     (4) presence of colostrum

     (5) signs of inflammation

       (a) heat

       (b) redness

       (c) pain

   b) intervention

     (1) ice packs to relieve engorgement

     (2) soothing ointments to prevent nipple cracking

     (3) breasts should be supported with well fitting bra

       (a) nipple at midline

       (b) no downward or upward pressure on breasts

       (c) if engorgement is so severe that baby cannot feed, milk should be manually expressed

     (4) nipples should be cleansed without soap

     (5) any sign of infection or inflammation should be reported to physician

8. abdomen

   a) assessment

     (1) mother should raise her head and shoulders while lying flat in bed with legs extended

     (2) nurse can then assess the width of the diastasis recti (separation of muscles at middle of abdomen)

   b) intervention

     (1) chin-raising postpartum exercise will help to strengthen abdominal muscles

     (2) woman lies on back and slowly raises head and tries to put chin on her chest. Head is raised to a count of four and lowered to count of four. Both head and shoulders may be raised as progress is made in the exercise

9. vital signs

   a) assessment

     (1) temperature: may rise slightly after delivery due to dehydration

        (a) any temperature of 100.4°F, for two successive days after the first postpartum day may be an untoward symptom

    (2) pulse
        (a) bradycardia may occur, usually between 60 and 70
            1. caused by decreased cardiac output
            2. hydremia
        (b) tachycardia
            1. may be caused by difficult labor
            1. may indicate hemorrhage, shock, or illness
    (3) blood pressure
        (a) should remain normal
        (b) hypotension may occur after saddle block
        (c) if elevated, may be sign of complications
        (d) hypertension may be a sign of preeclampsia
        (e) moderate elevation of blood pressure may occur from use of ergotrate or excitement

  b) nursing intervention
    (1) frequent monitoring of all vital signs immediately after delivery
    (2) routine observation during subsequent period
    (3) careful observation will help prevent or detect complications

10. nutrition
  a) assessment
    (1) weight loss after delivery
    (2) intake of nutrients
        (a) increased need for protein and vitamins
            1. aids in repair of tissue and healing process
        (b) increased iron intake
            1. aids in restoring blood to its normal state
    (3) may have postanesthesia nausea and vomiting
    (4) nutritional status
        (a) skin color and turgor
        (b) overweight or underweight
        (c) excessive fatigue
        (d) signs of vitamin deficiencies
        (e) hemoglobin and hematocrit lab reports
    (5) cultural dietary patterns
    (6) knowledge of nutrition
    (7) usual eating habits
    (8) economic resources to meet nutritional needs
  b) intervention
    (1) immediately after delivery
        (a) if nausea occurs
            1. prevent aspiration
            2. limit fluid intake
            3. medications as ordered
            4. mouth care essential
            5. ice chips to relieve thirst

             (b) monitor parental fluid intake
- (2) provide a diet that is nutritionally adequate and meets the cultural patterns and eating habits of the client
- (3) teach nutrition as indicated by assessment
- (4) assist in budgetary planning to meet nutritional needs
- (5) if anemia is present
  - (a) conserve patient energy
  - (b) provide food high in iron
  - (c) iron and vitamin supplements may be ordered
- (6) nutritional counselling for obesity or underweight
11. ambulation is now permitted within an hour after delivery. Observe for signs of weakness or fainting

C. Assessment and intervention relating to mothering role
1. assessment
  a) reaction to labor and delivery
    - (1) excitement or depression
    - (2) anger and hostility
    - (3) fears
    - (4) change in husband-wife relationship
    - (5) mother-child interaction
  b) puerperal restoration
    - (1) dependency needs
    - (2) learning needs
      - (a) knowledge of infant and child care
      - (b) cultural values relating to child-rearing
        - 1. father's role
      - (c) economic factors
      - (d) community resources
      - (e) parents' level of ability to understand and assimilate instruction
    - (3) initiative
    - (4) assumption of mothering role
    - (5) readiness for discharge
      - (a) available assistance in the home for new mother and child
      - (b) plans for child care
    - (6) parental adjustment to new role
      - (a) identify maladjustment cues
        - 1. unhappiness over sex or appearance of baby
        - 2. doesn't talk about baby
        - 3. doesn't touch or look at baby
        - 4. calls baby it
2. intervention
  a) taking-in process
    - (1) patient allowed to be dependent
    - (2) should not be rushed in taking over responsibility for own care and care of baby
    - (3) encourage verbalization of delivery experience and of fears and anxieties

    b) taking hold phase
       (1) constant reassurance and encouragement in mothering role
       (2) avoid fatigue in care of baby
       (3) allow mother to assume initiative in care of self and baby
       (4) optimum time for instruction
    c) going home
       (1) instruction given for care of self
          (a) postpartal examination
          (b) personal hygiene
          (c) sexual activity
          (d) information regarding reestablishment of menstrual cycle and fertility
          (e) importance of avoiding fatigue and muscle strain
       (2) instruction relating to child care
          (a) importance of continuing health care and supervision
          (b) physical care of infant
          (c) information regarding normal growth and development
          (d) safety precautions
          (e) feeding techniques
    d) parental child bonding
       (1) parental feelings may take time to develop after the birth of the first child
       (2) the work of Klaus and Kennell (maternal-infant bonding) emphasizes the importance of providing opportunities immediately after birth for the development of bonding or attachment behaviors between parents and baby
       (3) early and prolonged contact between parents and baby has a positive effect on parent-infant bonding
       (4) being present at the birth of their baby increases attachment behavior
       (5) parents have common ways of responding to their new babies
          (a) mothers usually touch and fondle their infants in the "en face" position, making eye contact with them and talking to them
          (b) the response of the infant with body or eye movements to the mother's attachment behavior strengthens the bonding process
          (c) fathers who handle their infants with close eye and skin contact soon after the birth also strengthen paternal attachment behaviors
          (d) parents who are responding to the recent loss of another child or loved person may have difficulty with early bonding

        (e) parents who have high anxiety over their infants right after birth may continue to be anxious as the child grows and develops

        (f) some parents take longer to develop bonding behaviors than others even with early contact

        (g) a high state of alertness in mother and infant increases attachment behaviors immediately after birth (Klaus and Kennell, 1976)

(6) early parental bonding may be a factor in the prevention of child abuse

(7) new parents should be informed of the normality of lack of immediate strong feelings towards the child

(8) facilitation of parental bonding can be accomplished by

        (a) allowing mother to examine and touch her undressed child

        (b) following delivery encourage parents to spend time in close contact with the newborn; immediate breast feeding is encouraged

           1. if mother has been anesthesized, safety precautions must be observed

        (c) allow mother to verbalize her concerns and questions

        (d) point out positive factors about baby's adjustment and progress

        (e) provide positive reinforcement of mother's mothering activities

        (f) primiparas need detailed instruction and repetition of child care activities. All mothers need support and encouragement

        (g) rooming-in provides an optimum situation for bonding

        (h) stay with mother during feeding time if anxiety is present

        (i) provide father with an opportunity to verbalize feelings about child and assist him in carrying out child care activities. Give positive reinforcement

e) parents should be counselled about the possibility of postpartal blues occurring after discharge from hospital

(1) the transitory nature of phenomenon should be explained

(2) knowledge of the possibility of having ambivalent feelings about the baby should be explained to parents to prevent guilt feelings from occurring

(3) husband and family should be aware of the importance of providing assistance to the mother to prevent helplessness and overwhelming responsibility

III.   DRUGS USED DURING POSTPARTAL PERIOD

A.   Oxytocic drugs are usually given immediately after delivery
     by injection or IV and for several days postpartum.  They are
     given orally to assist in involution by stimulating uterine con-
     tractions
     1. ergonovine maleate (Ergotrate) 1/320 g
     2. methylergonovine maleate (Methergine) is a synthetic form
        of Ergotrate; dosage is usually 1/320 g
     3. drugs may increase intensity of after-pains and also may
        elevate blood pressure

B.   Lactation suppressants inhibit pituitary from secreting pro-
     lactin by raising estrogen blood level.  All antilactogenic
     drugs should be given as soon as possible after delivery
     1. deladumone is a long-acting estrogen-androgen combina-
        tion that is given immediately after delivery by injection;
        only one dose is needed
     2. stilbestrol and diethylstilbestrol are examples of synthetic
        estrogens which are administered by mouth as soon after
        delivery as possible.  The usual dosage is 5 mg.  Head-
        ache, vomiting and dizziness are rare side effects

C.   Analgesics are used as necessary to ease the discomfort of
     after-pains or perineal soreness.  Darvon is most commonly
     used and is usually given in 32 or 65 mg doses and adminis-
     tered orally

D.   Sedatives: many sedative preparations have been used to as-
     sist the patient in sleeping.  Sedatives should be avoided be-
     cause of their adverse effect on the sleep cycle

E.   Antibiotics may be prescribed to control any infection that
     may occur.  Dosage and preparation used varies with organ-
     ism responsible for infection

F.   In breast feeding mothers, medications should be used with
     extreme caution as they enter the milk supply

# CHAPTER 17

BREAST FEEDING

I.   ANATOMY OF THE BREAST

A.   Composition
1. internal
   a) glandular tissue
   b) fat
   c) each breast contains 15-20 lobes connected by fibrous tissues and fatty walls
      (1) lobes subdivided into lobules
      (2) lobules contain acini cells
         (a) milk secretion originates in acini cells
         (b) capillaries in acini cells filter essential elements needed for milk production from blood, by osmosis
   d) duct structure
      (1) duct network carries milk from lobule to lobe to nipple
      (2) lactiferous sinuses and ducts form reservoirs for milk storage
         (a) located near nipple
2. external
   a) covered by skin
   b) areola
      (1) surrounds nipple
      (2) color varies with skin tone
         (a) darkens with pregnancy
      (3) contains montgomery glands which are sebaceous glands that enlarge during pregnancy

B.   Nipple
1. erectile tissue
2. contains milk duct openings

C.   Size of breast does not affect lactation ability

II.   PHYSIOLOGY

A.   During pregnancy
1. rapid development of glandular tissue
   a) because of estrogen levels

2. glandular tissue becomes secreting cells
   a) because of progesterone levels
3. lactogenic hormone (prolactin) inhibited by estrogen and progesterone until after birth, thereby preventing milk production
4. colostrum production begins during second trimester of pregnancy

B. Establishment of lactation
   1. decreased levels of estrogen and progesterone after delivery cause pituitary to secrete lactogenic hormone
   2. colostrum secretion increases and provides adequate nourishment until milk production on the third day
      a) milk production may be preceded by engorgement lasting 24-48 hours

C. Mechanisms of breast feeding
   1. sucking activates nerve impulses from nipple to spinal cord, to pituitary gland
      a) anterior pituitary produces prolactin only if breasts are emptied
      b) posterior pituitary secretes oxytocin causing "let down" reflex, causing milk to be ejected from ducts
         (1) oxytocin stimulated by sound of baby's cry or sucking
         (2) oxytocin inhibited by fright or stress
   2. successful breast feeding depends on adequate production of prolactin and oxytocin
   3. emotional factors significantly affect lactation by inhibiting hormone production

III. EFFECT OF LACTATION ON THE MOTHER

A. Physiological
   1. increased stress on metabolic system
   2. increased need for calcium and phosphate
      a) if intake is not adequate, calcium and phosphates will be drawn from mother's skeletal system, weakening bones
      b) usually a large amount of calcium and phosphate is stored in mother's bones, so only a poorly nourished mother will have difficulty
   3. increase of dental cavities not related to calcium deficiency during lactation, but rather, to enhanced bacterial growth in mouth
   4. involution is assisted
   5. decreased incidence of breast cancer
   6. engorgement less painful

B. Psychological
   1. number of mothers who breast feed is related to social and cultural factors
      a) success or failure in breast feeding depends largely on emotional factors and attitudes
   2. nursing is a pleasurable experience if the mother is ready and accepting
   3. aversions to breast feeding can be caused by
      a) sexual inhibitions
      b) dislike of nudity
      c) fear of loss of figure
      d) unpleasant previous breast feeding experiences
      e) difficult or unpleasant labor
      f) lack of support and instruction by health personnel
      g) leakage of breasts
      h) lack of freedom
   4. positive reactions to breast feeding
      a) faster development of maternal feeling
      b) economical
      c) time-saving (no preparation of formula)
      d) feeling of fulfillment of completion of maternal cycle
      e) there has been a steady increase in the number of breast-feeding mothers since the middle 1960s

IV. BENEFITS OF BREAST-FEEDING TO THE NEWBORN

A. Each 100 ml of milk contains 75 kcal
   1. fat makes up largest calorie component
   2. lactose provides main CHO source; metabolizes to glucose and galactose for energy
      a) promotes growth of lactobaccilli which acts to control growth of harmful bacteria in intestine
      b) lactose enhances absorption of calcium needed to prevent rickets
   3. protein-amino acids, cystine and taurine, found in high levels in human milk and low levels in cow's milk may stimulate tissue and brain growth
   4. proteins found in abundance in human milk are more easily digested than casein proteins which are higher in cow's milk

B. Renal solute load on kidney of breast-fed infant is much lower than the formula-fed infant

C. Breast milk contains many antiinfective ingredients such as interferon, leucocytes, immunoglobulins

D. Breast milk does not contain food antigens that are present in cow's milk, thereby minimizing potential allergies

V.   NURSING IMPLICATIONS

A.   Need for instruction, support and encouragement

B.   Nurses' attitudes may affect outcome

C.   Medications
     1. syntocin: synthetic oxytocin administered by nasal spray
        to activate let-down reflex
     2. any estrogen preparation is contraindicated

D.   Care of breasts
     1. support with bra or binder
        a) nipple at midline
        b) no pressure exerted downward or upward
        c) garment should give good support, but not be too tight
     2. wash breasts daily, no soap on nipples
     3. careful inspection of nipples for cracks or soreness
     4. observation of breasts for mastitis
     5. pads in bras to absorb leakage
     6. prevention of nipple damage
        a) new research indicates that the practice of limiting
           nursing time during initial breast feedings does not pre-
           vent nipple soreness. Mothers should be instructed to
           use both breasts and to allow baby to feed until it is sat-
           isfied to stimulate the supply/demand response. The
           mother should be careful that pressure is not placed on
           one part of the areola and that as much of the areola as
           possible is placed into the baby's mouth
        b) baby should be put to breast immediately after delivery
           and at frequent intervals thereafter whenever the baby
           is hungry (Riordan and Countryman, 1980)
     7. prevention of engorgement
        a) if breast is not completely emptied, manual expression
           of remainder of milk should be used to relieve engorge-
           ment. It can also be used to provide a relief bottle for
           the nursing mother once the milk supply is well estab-
           lished
           (1) after washing hands, client cups breast in her hand
               and places thumb and forefinger together behind nip-
               ple, and applies pressure toward chest wall
           (2) pressing and releasing should be done rythmically
               to release milk flow
           (3) milk should be directed into a container
     8. when releasing infant from breast, break vacuum around
        nipple by insertion of finger between baby's mouth and
        breast
     9. air drying after feeding
    10. position baby correctly at level of breast
    11. use of vitamin or lanolin ointment

E.   Maintaining milk supply
1. do not feed baby supplementary bottles during early period of lactation until milk is well established
2. alternate breasts for each feeding to allow complete emptying after milk supply is established
3. if baby fails to empty breast, teach mother manual expression of milk
4. feed baby on demand schedule
5. if soreness occurs use nipple shield

F.   Mother assisted to find most comfortable feeding position

G.   Nutrition
1. increase caloric intake 600-1000 calories daily according to individual need
2. protein increased to 20 g daily
3. increased intake of calcium, iron, vitamins A, C, and D
4. increased fluid intake
5. foods to be avoided
   a) foods causing allergic reactions in infants such as chocolate, etc.
   b) foods causing gaseous reactions in infants
6. drug intake must be monitored by physician

VI.   CONTRAINDICATIONS TO BREAST FEEDING

A.   Chronic debilitating diseases

B.   Communicable diseases

# CHAPTER 18

COMPLICATIONS OF THE POSTPARTUM PERIOD

I. ONE OF THE OBJECTIVES OF NURSING CARE DURING THE POSTPARTAL PERIOD IS TO PREVENT POTENTIAL COMPLICATIONS AND TO LIMIT THEIR EFFECT IF THEY DO OCCUR

II. POSTPARTUM HEMORRHAGE

A. Definition
1. bleeding from birth canal in excess of 500 ml
2. delayed postpartum hemorrhage may occur up to 2 weeks after delivery
   a) breast feeding decreases incidence

B. Normal blood loss during and after delivery is 50-300 ml

C. Hemorrhaging occurs in 5% of deliveries

D. Etiology
1. uterine atony (90% of cases)
2. vaginal and cervical lacerations
3. retention of placental fragments, clotting defects
4. low or absent fibrinogen in blood
5. distention of bladder

E. Predisposing factors
1. controllable causes
   a) operative deliveries
      (1) forceps
      (2) injuries
   b) deep anesthesia
      (1) relaxation of abdominal muscles
   c) prolonged labor and maternal exhaustion
   d) mismanagement of third stage of labor
      (1) kneading and squeezing of uterus may cause incomplete placental separation
   e) internal podalic version: changing the fetal position through manual manipulation through vagina (rarely utilized in modern obstetrics)
2. predetermined and uncontrollable causes

        a) overdistention of uterus
          (1) multiple pregnancy
          (2) hydramnios
          (3) large size baby
             (a) if baby weighs 3200 g or more
             (b) 4000 g or more weight: one in two chance of bleeding
        b) abruptio placenta
        c) placenta previa
        d) history of previous postpartum hemorrhage
        e) blood dyscrasias

F.    Symptoms
    1. bleeding may be moderate, continuous and steady
        a) extent of blood loss may not be realized
        b) vital signs may not immediately indicate the seriousness of blood loss
    2. bleeding may be massive and intense
        a) vital signs reflect amount of blood loss
          (1) pulse rapid and thready
          (2) pallor
          (3) falling blood pressure
          (4) chilliness
          (5) dyspnea and air hunger
        b) restlessness
        c) disturbed vision
        d) unconsciousness

G.    Diagnosis
    1. condition of fundus
        a) boggy fundus may be indication of uterine atony
        b) fundus firm and contracted rules out uterine atony, but indicates need for search in vaginal and cervical area for lacerations
    2. bright red blood is usually due to lacerations
    3. venous blood is usually from the uterus
    4. blood should be checked for fibrinogen levels
        a) afibrinogenemia may be cause of hemorrhage
        b) afibrinogenemia may result from hemorrhage

H.    Prognosis
    1. depends upon mother's health status before and during labor; if following conditions exist, prognosis is not as favorable
        a) anemia
        b) exhaustion from prolonged labor
        c) poor uterine muscle tone
        d) poor nutritional status

I.   Treatment
    1. during third stage
        a) if severe blood loss occurs before placental delivery
            (1) fundal pressure
                (a) not squeezing or kneading
            (2) manual removal of placenta
                (a) if placenta accreta is present, attempts to re-
                    move placenta manually may cause massive hem-
                    orrhage
    2. after third stage
        a) uterine atony
            (1) oxytocin administered
            (2) bimanual uterine compression
            (3) fluid, blood and fibrinogen replacement
            (4) hysterectomy if all else fails
        b) lacerations of cervix and vagina
            (1) repair
            (2) sulcus tear even if repaired is prone to hemorrhage
            (3) packing of vagina

J.   Nursing care
    1. assessment for prevention
        a) careful monitoring of
            (1) vital signs
            (2) uterine tone
            (3) amount and character of bleeding
    2. intervention for prevention
        a) correct technique in use of uterine massage
            (1) avoid overstimulation
        b) oxytocics given as ordered
    3. assessment during hemorrhage
        a) save blood stained linen to aid in determining amount of
           blood loss
        b) vital signs monitored
        c) observe fluid and electrolyte balance
        d) check for transfusion reactions
    4. intervention during hemorrhage
        a) maintain bladder tone when vaginal packing is used
            (1) encourage voiding
            (2) increase fluid intake
            (3) catheterize if necessary
        b) strict asepsis since resistance to infection is lower
        c) nutrition: added protein, iron and vitamin C
        d) careful and progressive ambulation to prevent recur-
           rence

III. PUERPERAL INFECTION

A.   Definition
    1. any temperature of $100.4^{\circ}$ occurring in any two successive
       days in first 10 postpartal days except for first 24 hours

B.  Factors in control of incidence
    1. aseptic obstetrical technique
    2. increased prenatal care
    3. general improvement in health status and nutrition
    4. improved management of labor and delivery
    5. use of antibiotics

C.  Causative organisms
    1. most common: anerobic streptococcus
       a) normal flora of vagina, usually nonpathogenic
    2. beta hemolytic streptococcus
    3. staphylococcus
       a) may have become resistant to antibiotics
    4. E. coli
    5. gonococcus
    6. B. Welchi: rare, but occurs in criminal abortions
       a) associated with high mortality rate

D.  Predisposing factors
    1. hemorrhage and trauma during delivery
    2. exhaustion
    3. retention of placenta
    4. pre-existing condition can cause normal flora of vagina to
       become pathogenic
       a) anemia
       b) malnutrition
       c) debilitation

E.  Modes of infection
    1. droplet
    2. poor asepsis
    3. poor personal hygiene
    4. sexual relations after membranes rupture
    5. during vaginal examination, normal flora may be carried
       to uterus where they are pathogenic

F.  Types of infection
    1. local lesion of perineum, vagina, cervix, and endometrium
    2. local infection may extend through venous circulation to
       cause
       a) infectious thrombophlebitis
       b) septicemia
    3. local infection may extend through lymphatics to cause
       a) peritonitis: inflammation of the peritoneum
       b) parametritis: inflammation of the connective tissue sur-
          rounding the uterus
       c) salpingitis: inflammation of the fallopian tubes

G.  Symptoms, treatment and prognosis
    1. infections of perineum, vulva, vagina, and cervix

    a) symptoms
       (1) redness
       (2) swelling
       (3) pain
       (4) sensation of heat
       (5) serous and/or purulent discharge
       (6) burning and urination
       (7) temperature usually below 101°F
    b) treatment
       (1) opening and draining of wound
       (2) local application of antiseptic
       (3) antibiotic therapy
       (4) wet compresses
       (5) sitz baths
       (6) heat lamp
    c) prognosis
       (1) good if treatment begins before spread upwards
2. endometritis
    a) symptoms
       (1) discharge may either be foul smelling, profuse, or
           lochia may be retained, and discharge scant
       (2) temperature range 101°F to 105°F
          (a) chilling may accompany temperature rise
       (3) pulse and respiration rapid
       (4) uterus usually enlarged
          (a) involution disturbed
       (5) tenderness over uterus
       (6) after pains severe and prolonged
       (7) headache
       (8) insomnia
       (9) anorexia
     (10) milk secretion suppressed
    b) prognosis
       (1) if localized, usually recovers in 10 days
    c) treatment
       (1) antibiotics
       (2) bedrest: semi-Fowlers position
       (3) supportive therapy
       (4) increase fluid intake
       (5) aseptic precautions
3. infectious thrombophlebitis
    a) occurs in uterine, ovarian, hypogastric, femoral, pop-
       liteal, and saphenous veins
    b) symptoms
       (1) severe chills
       (2) swings in temperature: 96° to 105°F
       (3) pain, tenderness, redness, or blanching, heat or
          cold over site of superficial vein
       (4) deep veins: pain may be only visible symptom
    c) treatment

          (1) bedrest
          (2) antibiotics
          (3) hot soaks
          (4) anticoagulant therapy
          (5) observation for occurrence of embolism

       d) prognosis
          (1) good if no embolism occurs
          (2) embolism may cause death if it blocks a vital organ
          (3) recovery may be prolonged

    4. peritonitis
       a) symptoms
          (1) chill
          (2) fever $103^{o}$-$105^{o}$
          (3) pulse: very rapid, weak, compressable
          (4) excruciating pain
          (5) diarrhea and vomiting
          (6) furred tongue
          (7) restlessness
       b) treatment
          (1) antibiotics
          (2) supportive therapy
       c) prognosis
          (1) good to poor depending on early detection and treatment

H.   Nursing care
    1. assessment
       a) vital signs
       b) abnormal vaginal discharge (purulent)
          (1) foul odor
          (2) color
          (3) amount: scanty discharge may indicate an infectious process
       c) pain, redness, or swelling of the perineum
       d) sensation of heat
       e) discharge around suture line
       f) delayed involution
       g) pain and tenderness over uterus
       h) restlessness
       i) lethargy
       j) anorexia
    2. intervention
       a) maintain asepsis to prevent infection
          (1) teach mother proper techniques for handwashing, breast care and perineal care
       b) if infection occurs
          (1) continued and careful assessment
       c) isolation if necessary
          (1) if mother is isolated encouragement and support is essential

        (a) reports on baby's condition
        (b) family should be taught aseptic techniques so they
           can visit
     (2) mother should be encouraged to verbalize her feel-
       ings about her illness
     (3) maintain an increased fluid intake
     (4) encourage a high-protein diet
     (5) provide frequent, uninterrupted rest periods
     (6) give medication as ordered

IV.   NONINFECTIOUS THROMBOPHLEBITIS

A.    Causes
     1. venous stasis
       a) early ambulation has led to a decrease in incidence
     2. clotting defects
     3. excess fibrinogen

B.    Symptoms
     1. phlebothrombosis: spontaneous intravascular clotting with
       minimal inflammation
       a) may have no symptoms
       b) pain
       c) edema
       d) elevated T.P.R.
       e) dorsiflexion of foot causes pain in calf (Homan's sign)
       f) may lead to pulmonary embolism
     2. thrombophlebitis: inflammation of venous wall and clotting
       a) chill
       b) high fever
       c) pain
       d) edema
       e) bluish white color

C.    Treatment
     1. anticoagulants
     2. ace bandage to affected leg
     3. bedrest with leg elevated
     4. hot soaks

D.    Nursing care
     1. prevention
       a) early ambulation
       b) prevent stasis in leg circulation
         (1) proper use of stirrups
         (2) avoid prolonged sitting
     2. assessment of
       a) signs of inflammation and level of edema
       b) reaction to medication
         (1) evidence of increased bleeding

      c) reaction to immobility
      d) level of pain
      e) fear and anxiety level
   3. intervention
      a) never massage as clot becomes dislodged
      b) maintain bedrest with leg elevated
      c) maintain fluid intake
      d) hot soaks to affected leg as ordered
      e) deep breathing exercise and frequent position change prevent further complications
      f) encouragement and reassurance since hospitalization may be prolonged
      g) instruction to prevent reoccurence
      h) allow verbalization

## V. BREAST DISORDERS

A. Mastitis: inflammation or infection of breast
   1. symptoms
      a) usually occurs between first to fourth week postpartum
      b) engorgement of breast
      c) chills
      d) rise in T.P.R.
      e) breast hard, red and painful
   2. etiology
      a) infection through fissured nipples or organisms in lactiferous ducts
      b) most common organism: Staphylococcus aureus
      c) baby's throat source of infection
      d) may come from hospital personnel carriers
   3. prevention
      a) prevent cracked nipples
      b) wash nipples with plain water to prevent milk encrustation
      c) careful monitoring of hospital personnel for carriers
      d) if cracked nipples occur
         (1) apply A & D ointment or tincture of benzoin
         (2) omit nursing on affected side
         (3) manually express milk
   4. treatment
      a) antibiotics
      b) hot soaks
   5. prognosis
      a) usually good and clears rapidly

B. Breast abscess: localized, walled off infection
   1. may need incision if no response to treatment

C. Nursing care
   1. assessment

        a) condition of breast
           (1) pain
           (2) redness
           (3) heat
           (4) engorgement
        b) condition of nipples
        c) vital signs
        d) nursing or nonnursing mother
   2. intervention
        a) support breast
        b) prevention and treatment of cracked nipples
        c) medications: antibiotics and analgesia as ordered
        d) hot soaks as ordered
        e) instruction regarding aseptic techniques to prevent spread of infection
        f) nursing may be continued with consent of physician
        g) additional support and reassurance will be necessary since nursing may be painful

## VI. INFECTIONS COMMON DURING POSTPARTUM

A. Urinary tract
   1. prevented by
        a) aseptic technique in catheterization
        b) not allowing bladder to become distended
        c) if retention occurs, urine is removed
        d) proper instruction regarding perineal care and handwashing
   2. dilation of ureters - during pregnancy and trauma during delivery may predispose mother to urinary infections
   3. treated with antibiotics

B. Pneumonia
   1. incidence drastically lower since advent of early ambulation
   2. treated with antibiotics

## VII. HEMATOMAS

A. Symptoms
   1. severe local pain
   2. appearance of a tense, sensitive, and discolored tumor on the perineum
   3. if hematoma is in vagina and large, patient may not be able to void

B. Treatment
   1. ice packs as ordered
   2. small hematomas are left to absorb without treatment
   3. large hematomas may be incised and drained
        a) blood vessels are ligated if necessary

VIII. POSTPARTUM ECLAMPSIA

A.  If patient has a prenatal history of preeclampsia
    1. careful observation of blood pressure and renal output
    2. immediate reporting of symptoms indicating increasing
       severity of condition
    3. eclamptic convulsions may occur up to 1 week after de-
       livery
       a) blood pressure should return to normal within 2 weeks
    4. patient should be carefully followed for early detection of
       chronic hypertensive vascular disease

IX. POSTPARTUM PSYCHOSIS

A.  Occurs early and may be seen immediately postpartum

B.  Any of the classified psychoses may occur during the post-
    partum period

C.  Theoretical causes
    1. involution of pituitary which results in trophic hormone
       deficits (thyroid, adrenocortical, and gonadal)
    2. childbirth may act as acute stressor which precipitates a
       psychosis in a person prone to mental illness
       a) unable to withstand stress of labor and delivery
       b) future fear of coping with baby or changing role

D.  Signs and symptoms
    1. insomnia
    2. confusion
    3. irritability
    4. apathy and depression
    5. delusions and hallucinations
    6. delirium
    7. inappropriate affect

E.  Nursing care
    1. assessment
       a) presence of any of the signs and symptoms of psychoses
       b) negative reaction to baby or father of child

F.  Nursing implications
    1. reduce stress of labor and delivery for all mothers
       a) instruction
       b) natural childbirth if mother is adequately prepared and
          is capable
       c) father in labor room if prepared
       d) reassurance and emotional support
    2. anticipatory guidance to aid in transition to new role
    3. early detection of mothers who exhibit signs of problems
       with coping or adaptation to new role

4. care if symptoms occur
   a) careful observation and nursing care of mothers who exhibit signs of disorder
   b) do not leave symptomatic patients alone or without careful supervision because of high incidence of suicide
   c) immediate referral for psychiatric evaluation
   d) protect infant if safety is threatened

## STUDY QUESTIONS

1. What signs indicate that involution is progressing normally?
2. What are the symptoms of breast engorgement and their nursing implications?
3. What measures can be taken to relieve perineal discomfort?
4. What causes urinary problems during postpartal period?
5. What measures are used to suppress lactation?
6. How can the nurse assist the breast feeding mother?
7. What are pros and cons of breast feeding?
8. At second day postpartum what would constitute normal lochia? At tenth day?
9. What can be done to prevent postpartal constipation?
10. Differentiate between "postpartal blues" and "postpartal psychosis."
11. What are the predisposing factors that contribute to postpartal hemorrhage?
12. What measures should be taken to prevent postpartal infection?
13. What effect has early ambulation had on postpartal period?
14. How does care of patient with C/S differ from routine postpartum care?
15. What is the significance of the diuresis that occurs in postpartal period?
16. What is the significance of a rise in blood pressure during the postpartal period? A fall in pulse rate? A rise in temperature?
17. Differentiate between taking in and taking hold processes.
18. Why does breast feeding intensify after-pains?

## BIBLIOGRAPHY

Applebaum, R.: The Modern Management of Successful Breast Feeding, Pediatric Clinics of North America, Feb. 1970.

Branson, Helen: The Blind Mother, American Journal of Nursing, March, 1975.

Brown, M.S.: Preparation of the Breast for Breastfeeding, Nursing Research, pp. 448-451, Nov./Dec. 1975.

Clark, Ann and Affonso, Dyanne: Childbearing: A Nursing Perspective, F.A. Davis Co., Phila., 1979.

Countryman, B.: Hospital Care of the Breast-Fed Newborn, American Journal of Nursing, December, 1971.

Johnson, Joan Marie: Stillbirth - A Personal Experience, American Journal of Nursing, September, 1972.

Klaus, M. and Kenneth, J.: Human Maternal Behavior at First Contact with Her Young, Pediatrics, August, 1970.

Klaus, M.H. and Kennell, J.H.: Maternal-Infant Bonding. St. Louis, C.V. Mosby, 1976, pp. 1-60.

LeMasters, E.E.: Parenthood as a Crisis, in: Crisis Intervention: Selected Readings (H.J. Parad, ed.), New York, Family Association of America, 1965.

Liefer, Gloria: Rooming-In Despite Postpartal Complications, American Journal of Nursing, October, 1967.

Murdaugh, A. and Miller, L.: Helping the Breast-Feeding Mother, American Journal of Nursing, August, 1972.

Murdaugh, A. and Miller, L.: Physiology of Lactation, Population Reports, George Washington University Medical Center, Series J, No. 4, July, 1975.

Raphael, Dana: When Mothers Need Mothering, N.Y. Times Magazine, February 5, 1970.

Riordan, J. and Countryman, B.A.: Basics of Breastfeeding, JOGN Nursing, July/August and September/October, 1980, pp. 207-213, 273-283.

Rubin, Reva: Puerperal Change, Nursing Outlook, December, 1961.

Rubin, Reva: Basic Maternal Behavior, Nursing Outlook, November, 1961.

Schmitt, M.: Superiority of Breast Feeding: Fact or Fancy, American Journal of Nursing, July, 1970.

Seward, M. Elizabeth: Preventing Postpartum Psychosis, American Journal of Nursing, March, 1972.

Whitley, N.: Breast Feeding the Premature, American Journal of Nursing, September, 1970.

Whitley, N.: Preparation for Breastfeeding: A One-Year Follow-up of 34 Nursing Mothers, JOGN Nursing 7(3):44, May/June, 1978.

UNIT V: NEWBORN

CHAPTER 19

ANATOMY AND PHYSIOLOGY OF THE NEWBORN

I.  CIRCULATORY AND RESPIRATORY SYSTEMS

A.  Oxygenation of blood
    1. with first breath pulmonary circulation changes
        a) ductus arteriosus begins to atrophy and becomes liga-
           mentum arteriosum, blood is pumped into pulmonary
           artery by right ventricle
           (1) final closure from 3 weeks to 4 months
        b) more blood is returned from lungs to left atrium caus-
           ing pressure to rise and foramen ovale to close
           (1) placental circulation ceases
           (2) ends of hypogastric arteries atrophy and become
               known as hypogastric ligaments
           (3) ductus venosus becomes occluded and becomes the
               ligamentum venosum
           (4) umbilical vein becomes occluded and is known as
               ligamentum teres
    2. acrocyanosis (cyanosis of extremities) may be present for
       first 24 hours
    3. circumoral pallor may be present during feeding or cry-
       ing until foramen ovale is completely closed
    4. hypothrombinemia: prothrombin level is usually decreased
       after birth
        a) clotting time may be prolonged
        b) most acute between second and fifth day
        c) vitamin K is needed to produce prothrombin
           (1) spontaneous production of vitamin K is delayed until
               the normal flora of intestinal tract is established,
               usually within 1 week. Bacteria are needed to syn-
               thesize vitamin K in the intestine

II. PHYSIOLOGICAL RESILIENCE

A.  Neonate does not readily show overt signs and symptoms of
    abnormalities of body functioning such as
    1. body temperature variations (high or low)
    2. blood chemistry changes (i.e., glucose)
    3. changes in vital signs

B.  Disadvantages of physiological resilience
    1. conceals or minimizes physical signs of diagnostic value
    2. neonate does not react uniformly to drugs

C.  Advantages of physiological resilience
    1. when blood sugar drops for short periods the usually hypo-
       glycemic reaction does not occur: can tolerate fluctuations
       in blood chemistry with less damage than adults
    2. can survive without breathing longer than an adult and with
       less brain damage

III.  NEGATIVE BALANCE

A.  First few days of life neonate is in state of negative balance
    1. postnatal weight loss
    2. loss of body fluids
    3. decreases in
       a) hemoglobin after 2nd day
       b) nitrogen
       c) sodium
       d) chloride

B.  Positive balance is usually restored in 3-5 days

IV.  HEAT REGULATION

A.  Unstable heat regulatory system due to immature hypothala-
    mus
    1. with exposure to cold infant increases rate of metabolism
       without visible shivering
    2. neonate uses a metabolic process called NST (nonshivering
       thermogenesis) to produce heat. This increased metabo-
       lism uses up energy and oxygen. The heat that the infant
       manufactures during NST comes from brown fat metabo-
       lism. Brown fat is found in infants and when the available
       fat is used up the infant has difficulty maintaining body tem-
       perature when exposed to cold

B.  Body temperature greatly influenced by environment tempera-
    ture
    1. when external factors cause the amount of heat lost to ex-
       ceed the metabolic ability of the infant to maintain heat bal-
       ance, body temperature drops
       a) factors contributing to imbalance in heat regulation
          (1) air conditioned delivery rooms
          (2) immediate bathing of infant with prolonged and un-
              necessary body exposure
          (3) exposure during newborn physical assessment
    2. ability to maintain heat balance is also affected by the over
       heating of the environment

a) factors
   (1) overdressing
   (2) nursery temperature too high
   (3) incubator or infant warmer temperature too high

V. VITAL SIGNS

A. Temperature unstable (97°-98.6°)
   1. at birth slightly higher than mother's
   2. drops immediately after birth in adjustment to room temperature
   3. rises to normal in eight hours
   4. between second and fourth day there may be a temperature rise due to dehydration
      a) any temperature of 100°F that persists for more than 24 hours must be checked

B. Pulse
   1. rapid
   2. normal range: 120-150/minute
   3. irregular due to immature cardiac regulatory center in medulla

C. Respiration
   1. irregular in depth, rate, and rhythm
   2. normal range: 35-50/minute
   3. quiet
   4. synchronous: diaphragm and abdominal muscles rise together
   5. touching and stroking increases respiration and oxygen intake
   6. too vigorous suctioning at birth may lead to secondary apnea

D. Blood pressure
   1. 80/46 at birth, rising to 100/50 at 10 days
   2. difficult to get accurate reading
   3. a 1 in. cuff is used

VI. LENGTH AND MEASUREMENTS OF BODY

A. Length
   1. range: 19-21.5 in.
   2. males usually longer than females

B. Weight
   1. range: 6-8.5 lbs (2700-3850 g)
   2. girls usually weigh less than boys
   3. under 2500 g classified as premature and/or low birth weight

4. during first few days after birth, baby loses 6-10 oz (5-10% of birth weight) because of
   a) withdrawal of maternal hormones
   b) loss of fluid
   c) loss of meconium and urine
   d) usual NPO routine (12-24 hours)

C. Measurements
   1. head
      a) large in proportion to rest of body
      b) normal circumference 13.2-14.8 in
         (1) over 14.8 in may be hydrocephalic
         (2) under 13.2 in may be either microcephalic or premature
      c) fontanels
         (1) openings at point of union of skull bones
         (2) anterior fontanel is diamond shaped and is located at juncture of two parietal bones and two frontal bones
            (a) closes between 12 and 18 months
         (3) posterior fontanel
            (a) triangularly shaped opening between occipital and parietal bone
            (b) smaller than anterior fontanel
            (c) closes by end of second month
         (4) fontanels bulge when baby cries, strains or if there is intercranial pressure
         (5) depression of fontanel may occur during dehydration
   2. chest
      a) at birth has approximately same circumference as abdomen
      b) at 2 years chest circumference should exceed that of head

VII. SKIN

A. Dark pink

B. Soft

C. May be covered with lanugo and vernix caseosa
   1. vernix caseosa dries spontaneously
   2. lanugo disappears during first week of life

D. Desquamation (peeling)
   1. occurs during first 2-4 weeks

E. Milia: tiny white papillae
   1. obstruction of sebaceous glands particularly on nose and chin

F. Turgor
1. elasticity and fullness of subcutaneous tissue indicates state of hydration

G. Physiological jaundice (third to fifth day)
1. breakdown of excessive red blood cells no longer needed for oxygenation
2. liver unable to break down bilirubin as quickly as necessary
3. of no pathological significance
4. disappears between seventh and fourteenth day
5. when bilirubin levels rise above 15 mg/100 ml hyperbilirubinemia is present

VIII. GASTROINTESTINAL SYSTEM

A. Sucking pads in mouth and jaw disappear when baby no longer relies exclusively on sucking for food intake

B. Difficulty in moving solid food from lips to pharynx during first few months of life

C. Cardiac sphincter not fully developed at birth may cause baby to swallow excess amount of air. Burping alleviates discomfort

D. Stomach empties in 2 or 3 hours
1. slowed by foods high in protein and fat
2. demand feeding patterns respond to individual differences in digestive patterns

E. Stools
1. meconium
a) first fecal material
b) sticky, odorless, greenish-black in color
c) passed in 8-24 hours
(1) if no stool is passed within this time examination for obstruction is necessary
2. transitional
a) 3-5 days
b) loose, greenish yellow
c) contain mucus
3. stools after fifth day depend on feeding method
a) breast fed: yellow, soft, pleasant sourish odor; 2-4 per day
b) formula: light yellow, firm, unpleasant odor; 1-2 per day

IX. UMBILICAL CORD

A. Shrinks and darkens soon after birth

B. Turns black and complete necrosis occurs in 3-5 days

C. Falls off between 6-10 days

D. Heals completely within 2 weeks

X. ANOGENITAL AREA

A. Male
   1. penis and scrotum size varies
   2. testes descended in scrotal sacs
      a) undescended testes may remain in abdomen or inguinal canal and may require hormonal therapy or surgical intervention to correct
   3. foreskin of penis should be retractable
      a) phimosis: unretractable foreskin

B. Female
   1. labia majora not well developed
   2. labia minora appear large and are exposed
   3. genital area may be swollen and have blood tinged mucus discharge due to hormones transmitted by mother prenatally
      a) condition disappears in second or third week

XI. BREASTS

A. In both male and female, breasts may enlarge and secrete substance known as "witches milk"
   1. caused by hormones transferred by mother prenatally
   2. condition disappears in second or third week

XII. URINARY SYSTEM

A. Urine present in bladder at birth
   1. may void immediately or after several hours

B. Urine diluted because of immature kidney function

C. Voids frequently

XIII. SKELETAL SYSTEM

A. Bones soft and flexible

B. Joints elastic

C. Muscles are not strong, coordinated, or controlled
   1. can raise head slightly in prone position but not in supine
   2. cannot support own head when held in upright position

XIV. NERVOUS SYSTEM

A. Immature
   1. unstable
   2. poorly controlled
   3. sensitive to external stimuli

B. Important infant reflexes
   1. winking: occurs when something is brought near, or eyes are exposed to bright light
   2. coughing and sneezing: protective, clears respiratory tract
   3. yawning: infant takes in increased amounts of oxygen
   4. rooting: when infant's cheek is stroked, the head will turn in that direction, assisting him in locating nipple for feeding
   5. sucking: anything touching lips initiates sucking reflex
   6. gagging: protective mechanism to prevent aspiration
   7. grasp: any object placed in hands will be grasped
      a) grasping reflex fades with maturity and is replaced by conscious and purposeful movement
   8. walking reflex: when infant is held so that sole of foot touches a solid object, he will make walking motions
   9. moro (startle reflex): sudden stimulus causes infant to draw up legs, abduct and extend arms into embrace position
      a) stimulus may be sudden noise, movement, or abrupt change in position
      b) absence of a symmetrical moro response usually indicates an abnormality
   10. Babinski reflex: when sole of foot is stroked, toes flair outward. This response to the Babinski reflex is normal only in the infant
   11. tonic neck: when infant lies on back, his head will turn to one side and arm and leg on that side are extended, opposite arm and leg are flexed
   12. there are other infant reflexes that may be checked by physician

XV. SENSORY ABILITIES

A. Touch is most highly developed of all senses
   1. most acute on lips, tongue, ears, and forehead

B. Sight
   1. eyes blue-gray at birth and attain permanent color between third and sixth month
   2. pupils react to light
   3. bright lights appear to be unpleasant
   4. discrimination and recognition of objects develops with maturity

      5. strabismus and nystagmus may occur normally during first month

C.    Hearing
    1. immediate response to sounds
    2. by fourth week may recognize mother's voice
    3. reacts with Moro reflex to loud or sudden noises

D.    Taste
    1. more highly developed than sight or hearing

E.    Smell
    1. some infants appear to smell breast milk

XVI. SLEEP

A.    Neonate sleeps from 12-20 hours per day

B.    Awakened by internal discomfort, such as pain and hunger

XVII. IMMUNITY

A.    Some antibodies pass through placenta (i.e., measles, mumps, smallpox)

B.    Colostrum, in breast feeding mother, supplies antibodies

C.    Antibodies supply passive immunity for limited period of time

D.    High susceptibility to infection when antibodies are not present

# CHAPTER 20

## COMMON VARIATIONS OCCURRING IN THE NEWBORN

I. CEPHALOHEMATOMA

A. Collection of blood between cranial bone and periosteum

B. Caused by pressure of head against bony prominence of pelvis during labor
1. capillaries rupture under periosteum

C. May be apparent on delivery but may form up to second day of life

D. Characteristics
1. varying in size
2. firm to touch
3. increase in size for 1 or 2 days and then become softer

E. Regression of cephalohematoma usually occurs spontaneously during first 6 weeks of life

II. CAPUT SUCCEDANEUM

A. Swelling of soft tissues of presenting portion of scalp area encircled by cervix during labor

B. Apparent at birth

C. Subsides without treatment within 2 days

III. NEVUS FLAMMEUS

A. Nonelevated, irregularly shaped birth mark

B. Pink in color

C. Usually found
1. at base of neck
2. on eyelids
3. on upper lip

D.    Fades gradually and total regression usually occurs by the end of second year

IV.    FORCEPS MARKS

A.    Red or purplish bruises at site of forceps application

B.    Fade in a few days

V.    MOLDING

A.    Overlapping of cranial bones

B.    Results in irregularity and elongation of the head

C.    Caused by forcing of head through birth canal

D.    Most prevalent in first borns and after a long, difficult labor

E.    Returns to normal in a few days

F.    Molding may occur because of intrauterine pressure

VI.    SUBCONJUNCTIVAL HEMORRHAGE

A.    Red or purplish discoloration under conjunctiva

B.    Vary in size and are usually crescent shaped

C.    Caused by congestion and rupture of capillaries during birth

D.    Disappear within 1 or 2 weeks

VII.    CURTIS MARMORATA

A.    Pink or purplish capillary outlines on skin (mottling)

B.    Seen most over extremities

C.    Is thought to be vasomotor in origin

D.    Disappears when circulation is increased, transitory in nature

VIII.    MONGOLIAN SPOTS

A.    Nonelevated bluish-gray areas of pigmentation

B.    Seen most often in black, Asian, or Mediterranean infants

C.    Fade in early childhood

IX.   EDEMA OF SCROTUM

A.   Caused by pressure during labor and delivery

B.   Usually disappears in 2 weeks

X.   VARIATIONS IN SHAPE AND POSITION OF HEAD AND BODY

A.   Deviations from normal shape and position of head, face and extremities may occur because of position in utero

B.   Usually are self-correcting in early infancy

C.   Position of infant should be changed frequently to prevent permanent misshaping of head

## CHAPTER 21

## NURSING CARE OF THE NEWBORN

I.  ASSESSMENT

A.  Immediate evaluation of the newborn
    1. Apgar done 1 minute after birth and repeated in 5 minutes
        a) any baby with an Apgar below 7 should be considered a
           high risk infant
    2. gestational age assessment (Bash and Gold, 1981)
        a) important in differentiating between a premature baby
           and a baby who is small for gestational age (SGA) but is
           mature. It is also important to distinguish between the
           postmature baby and the baby who is large for gesta-
           tional age (LGA)
        b) classification categories
           (1) neonate at term: 38-42 weeks gestation
           (2) neonate born before term: less than 38 weeks gesta-
               tion
           (3) neonate born after term: after 42 weeks gestation
        c) assessment data used in determining gestational age in-
           cludes
           (1) weight: neonate may be average, below average or
               above average for gestational age based on weight
               percentile norms
           (2) measurements made during the pregnancy such as
               ultrasound scanning
           (3) physical and neurological signs of maturity
    3. careful monitoring is needed during the first and second
       reactive phases of the transition period of the newborn.
       During the second reactive phase suctioning of secretions
       may be necessary if they become profuse (Bash and Gold,
       1981)
        a) first reactive phase; immediately after birth: alert pe-
           riod, may have tachycardia and tachypnea
        b) after a period of several hours sleep the second reactive
           phase occurs usually followed by stability of pulse and
           respiration. Tachycardia and tachypnea may occur dur-
           ing the second reactive stage
    4. body inspection
        a) head
           (1) size of head checked to evaluate proportion between
               head and chest

216

        (a) circumference of head and chest recorded on newborn's chart

   (2) abnormalities in shape

        (a) molding

        (b) caput succedaneum

        (c) fontanels

           1. depression may indicate dehydration

           2. bulging may indicate hydrocephalus or neurological disorders

        (d) overriding of sutures

b) skin color

   (1) pallor may indicate shock or anemia

   (2) jaundice in first 48 hours may indicate hemolytic disease, liver, or biliary abnormality

        (a) early jaundice may be detected by placing several fingers on forehead or chest of baby and exerting gentle pressure; when fingers are suddenly removed, area will show a yellow tinge

   (3) cyanosis

        (a) acrocyanosis: normal phenomenon when rest of body is pink (first 24 hours)

        (b) circumoral pallor may indicate respiratory, cardiac, or neurological disease

        (c) when cyanosis decreases with crying, respiratory disorders should be suspected

        (c) when cyanosis increases with crying, heart disease is suspected

   (4) petechiae: pinpoint red spots due to ruptured capillaries, may indicate abnormality

   (5) purpura: bluish purplish discolorations caused by subdermal hemorrhage, may indicate abnormality or birth injury

c) skin conditions to be noted

   (1) rashes

   (2) redness

   (3) scratches

d) eyes

   (1) almond shape may indicate Down's syndrome

   (2) opacity may indicate congenital cataracts

   (3) discharges may indicate infection or injury

   (4) redness of conjunctiva may indicate injury or infection

        (a) isolation necessary if infection is present or suspected

e) ears

   (1) low abnormally shaped ears may indicate kidney malformation or chromosomal abnormality

   (2) the upper part of the ear lobe should be on same level as eye

f) mouth
   (1) asymmetry and abnormal contour may indicate paralysis
   (2) check for cleft palate and cleft lip
   (3) excessive salivation may indicate tracheo-esophageal fistula
   (4) check for tongue tie
   (5) check mucosa for abnormalities (i.e., white patches)
   (6) any of these conditions may hinder feeding
g) umbilical stump
   (1) check for three vessels, two arteries, and one vein
   (2) if three vessels are not present it may indicate congenital abnormalities
h) abdomen
   (1) check for distention
   (2) check for umbilical or diaphragmatic hernia
   (3) check for lack of synchrony between rise and fall of chest and abdomen during respirations. Movements should be synchronous
i) genitals and anal region
   (1) patency of anus may be tested by taking rectal temperature or by passage of meconium
   (2) condition of genital area should be checked for
      (a) swelling
      (b) phimosis
      (c) discharges
      (d) testes should be descended
      (e) presence of abnormalities
      (f) fissures or sores
j) skeletal system
   (1) symmetry of movement of extremities
   (2) check for dislocation of hip
      (a) abduct hips to frog position
      (b) check symmetry of buttock creases and length of legs
   (3) check number of fingers and toes
   (4) test for range of foot motion
      (a) dorsiflexion
      (b) dorsiflexion and inversion
      (c) dorsiflexion and eversion
      (d) plantar flexion and inversion
      (e) plantar flexion and eversion
      (f) plantar flexion
      (g) limitations of any of these movements should be reported
k) nervous system
   (1) neurological reflexes should be elicited to rule out neurological disorders
   (2) tremors, convulsions should be reported

5. vital signs
   a) respiration should be 40-60/minute, synchronous, without retractions
   b) temperature should remain in range of 97.5-98 (axillary) or $97^9$-$99^5$ rectal
   c) heart rate: normal range is 120-160 beats per minute, consistently slow or overly rapid rates may indicate circulatory problems. Rate rises during crying and drops during sleep

6. cry
   a) weak, shallow, high-pitched cry may indicate intracranial disorders
   b) grunting or moaning during breathing often accompanies respiratory distress
   c) stridor, a harsh, whistling sound, may indicate partial obstruction of respiratory tract
   d) wheezing may indicate abnormality
   e) cry resembling a cat's meow may indicate a mental retardation syndrome

B.   Continuing observation of newborn
1. color
2. cry
3. respiration
   a) excessive mucus may block respiratory passages
4. temperature
5. elimination
   a) should void within 24 hours
   b) voiding should be frequent
   c) meconium should be passed within 24 hours
   d) stools should be checked for abnormalities
6. sleeping
7. activity level
8. weight
9. feeding behavior and patterns
10. signs of infant distress
   a) increased rate and/or difficulty in respiration
   b) excessive mucus or drooling
   c) sternal retractions
   d) worried facial expressions
   e) cyanosis
   f) abdominal distention or mass
   g) inadequate voiding and/or expulsion of meconium
   h) vomiting of bile-stained fluid
   i) jaundice 24-48 hours after birth
   j) convulsions
11. Brazelton neonatal assessment scale may be used to assess the behavioral characteristics of the newborn and reflex patterns (Brazelton, 1973)
   a) nursing care can be planned to meet the needs of the infant based on individual behavior patterns

      b) parents can be taught to respond to their infant's needs through mapping of the baby's usual behavioral patterns and responses

      c) Brazelton scale is used to assess the behavioral responses of the infant within six states of alertness
        (1) sleep states
          (a) deep sleep
          (b) light sleep
        (2) awake states
          (a) semiasleep, drowsy
          (b) quiet alert
          (c) active alert
          (d) crying
        (3) seventeen reflex responses are also assessed (e.g., plantar grasp, hand grasp, Babinski, tonic neck, Moro, rooting, sucking and others)

## II. INTERVENTION

A. Maintenance of adequate oxygenation
1. airway of infant must remain patent
2. mucus in nose and mouth should be gently suctioned with a bulb syringe or nasal catheter
3. color and respirations must be carefully monitored. First 12 hours in newborn are particularly important for close observation
4. infant placed on side to prevent aspiration
5. care must be taken during feeding to prevent aspiration
6. monitor for periods of apnea (Glista, 1978)
    a) apnea may be defined as cessation of respiration for 15 seconds when accompanied by cyanosis, or heart rate under 100/minute and cessation of respiration for 20 seconds or more. Periodic breathing occurs commonly in newborns and is defined as respiratory pauses of 10-15 seconds without bradycardia or cyanosis
    b) severe or frequent periods of apnea is associated with morbidity and mortality
    c) factors causing apnea include respiratory problems, deep suctioning and stimulation of the posterior pharynx, high environmental temperature, metabolic disorders such as hypoglycemia, CNS disorders, sleep state and abnormal positions
    d) in uncomplicated apnea cutaneous stimulation such as stroking the skin will usually stimulate respirations
    e) in apnea associated with pathology the underlying condition must be treated along with the apnea

B. Nutrition
1. newborn usually NPO for 6-12 hours
2. glucose or water usually given as first feeding

3. if sucking, swallowing, and retention is normal, formula is started
4. breast fed babies need not be kept NPO because colostrum is nonirritating and easily swallowed even in the presence of excessive mucus and also provides antibodies
5. formulas
   a) calculated according to age and body weight
   b) composition
      (1) protein: less in human milk than any formula preparations
      (2) fat: more in human milk than in formula preparations
      (3) CHO: more in human milk than in most other preparations
      (4) formulas such as Similac and Enfamil, more closely approximate human milk composition than does evaporated milk
6. preparation of formulas
   a) sterilization by aseptic or terminal methods recommended when formula will be stored in refrigerator for 24 hours, to prevent bacterial contamination
7. feeding the formula fed baby
   a) demand feeding schedule is preferred
   b) hospital nursery routine is often based on 3-4 hour schedule and may interfere with demand feeding
   c) temperature of formula may be warmed to room temperature or given directly from refrigerator
   d) the usual amount taken by baby during first initial feedings is 1-1.5 oz
   e) amount of intake gradually increases until full amount is taken (approximately 3-4 oz)
   f) amount of intake varies with metabolic rate of individual baby
      (1) an active baby will usually require more calories than a placid one
   g) propping should be discouraged due to danger of aspiration and baby's need for close physical contact during feeding
   h) tilt bottle so that excessive air is not ingested during feeding
   i) nipple should be patent and openings small enough to permit slow feeding which allows sucking needs to be fulfilled and helps prevent tongue thrust (abnormal forward thrust of tongue during swallowing) which can lead to speech and/or orthodontic problems
      (1) a special nipple is available which simulates the same sucking mechanism used in breast feeding and is a preventive for tongue thrust (Nuk-Sauger nipple)
   j) baby should be burped during and after the feeding to allow air that has been swallowed to be expelled

       k) regurgitation and vomiting may occur due to
         (1) excessive mucus
         (2) improper feeding
         (3) abnormalities of GI tract
       l) stomach of newborn empties in 1-1/2-4 hours or more
      m) baby signals his hunger through crying

C. Positioning
1. normal attitude of newborn is one of flexion
2. when on back, the thighs are externally rotated and knees are slightly flexed
3. when in prone position the baby has the ability to turn head to side
4. baby should not be placed on back because of danger of aspiration
5. position should be changed frequently, alternating between right and left side and prone position
6. prevent hyperextension of neck

D. Maintaining body temperature
1. in order to protect the normal temperature of deep body tissues, external heat must be supplied
2. methods of maintaining normal temperature
   a) avoid exposure during bathing
   b) warm room temperature
   c) avoid drafts
   d) adequate clothing
3. excessive heat should be avoided
   a) in warm weather baby should be clothed appropriately
   b) room temperature should not be excessive

E. Safety
1. asepsis
   a) individual equipment
   b) adequate spacing of cribs, nursery should not be over-crowded
   c) rotation of nursery to which child is admitted
     (1) each unit is completely emptied and cleaned before another group is admitted
   d) nursery personnel limited in number
   e) medical asepsis is vital in nursery care of newborn
     (1) scrub gowns are worn by nursery personnel
     (2) hand washing
       (a) before entering nursery
       (b) between care of each baby
   f) cultures of various nursery areas taken at routine intervals
   g) dry dusting not utilized in terminal disinfection of equipment on discharge of baby
   h) immediate isolation when there is

(1) any suspicion of illness in baby
(2) an extramural birth
  i) if mother has a communicable disease, she should not feed baby
  j) diapers and waste should be placed in covered containers
  k) mothers should be taught aseptic practices
  l) personnel should not work in nursery when ill
2. mechanical safety
  a) never leave baby on flat surface unattended
  b) baby should be held securely with adequate head support at all times
  c) care should be taken when safety pins are used
  d) when baby is weighed he should be protected from falling
  e) thermometer should not be left in baby without supervision

F. Comfort measures
  1. bath
    a) frequency and value of sponge bathing in first week of life is debated
    b) genital area must be cleansed with each diaper change
      (1) girls' genitalia cleansed from front to back
    c) nonirritating soap should be used
    d) cord area left exposed
    e) tub bath given when umbilicus is healed
  2. clothing should be loose and unrestrictive
  3. flat, firm mattress without a pillow is best
  4. diapers should be changed frequently

G. Sleep and rest
  1. usually baby sleeps 12-20 hours daily
  2. sucking releases into sleep
  3. babies vary in sleep and activity patterns
  4. are usually awakened by hunger and/or discomfort

H. Circumcision
  1. removal of foreskin covering the glans penis
  2. indications
    a) phimosis: inability to retract foreskin
    b) done prophylactically to insure genital cleanliness
      (1) if foreskin is not retracted frequently during personal hygiene, smegma builds up and may cause irritation
    c) ritual of Hebrew religion
  3. timing of procedure is dependent upon
    a) condition of baby
      (1) delayed in babies with Rh factor, fetal distress, or other contraindications
    b) ritual or nonritual

        (1) ritual on eighth postpartum day
        (2) nonritual varies from time of birth to fourth day of
            life
    4. nursing implications
        a) dressing is not disturbed for 24 hours
        b) diaper area kept clean and dry
        c) watch for bleeding; report at once
        d) bathing delayed until area is healed

I.  Emotional needs of newborn
    1. sensory stimulation
        a) tactile, visual, and auditory stimulation are necessary
           to enhance the emotional, mental and physical develop-
           ment of the child
        b) sense of touch most developed sense at birth making
           cuddling, holding and stroking a particularly valuable
           form of stimulation
    2. mothering
        a) feeling of mothering transmitted to baby through his
           senses by the manner in which the baby is handled,
           spoken to and played with
        b) sense of trust developed through the manner in which
           the mother meets the needs that are being expressed by
           baby. The primary needs of the baby are feeding, re-
           lief of discomfort and anxiety and the need to be loved
            (1) in order to assist the mother in meeting the emo-
                tional needs of the infant an assessment of their in-
                teraction must be made
                (a) eye contact
                (b) the way baby is held
                (c) vocalization to child
                (d) touching and stroking behavior of mother
                (e) reaction of baby to mother
                    1. appears relaxed in mother's arms
                    2. stops crying when held by mother
                    3. becomes rigid
                    4. seem to cuddle into mother's arms
                (f) are there feeding problems?
                (g) is the mother anxious for baby to be returned to
                    nursery?
                (h) verbal and nonverbal signs of mother when baby
                    is present
                (i) mother's response to infant's crying
                (j) when father is present and is in contact with the
                    infant similar assessment can be made
    3. intervention
        a) if there are disturbed interactions noted between parents
           and child
            (1) encourage verbalization of feeling of inadequacy, fear
                and hostility related to infant care

(2) maintain a nonjudgemental attitude
(3) support the mother by reassurance, praise when indicated and teaching her aspects of child care that she is unsure of
(4) enlist a support system of friends, others in similar situations and relatives
(5) referral for further supervision and assistance if necessary
(6) assist mother in meeting her own dependency needs

J.  Learning needs of the mother in relation to care of the newborn child
1. for an adequate plan of teaching to be established it is necessary to assess the knowledge base and abilities of the new mother
    a) psychomotor skills of mother regarding feeding, handling, bathing, etc.
    b) knowledge of growth and development
    c) cultural practices and beliefs related to child-rearing
    d) motivation for learning
    e) level of ability to understand instruction
2. assessment must be made of mother's feelings toward the baby since anxiety and fear may interfere with learning
3. depending on the assessment the following learning opportunities should be provided
    a) an opportunity to practice under supervision the psychomotor skills such as feeding, bathing, dressing and handling, etc.
    b) preparation of the formula
    c) the relationship between usual child care practices and cultural beliefs
    d) nutrition for the developing infant
    e) safety needs for the baby
    f) importance of providing sensory stimulation to assist in development (all sensory modalities should be included)
    g) importance of consistency in caring patterns so that the child will know what to expect
    h) assistance in developing a flexible time framework within which the mother may work out a schedule which will meet family needs, self needs and infant's needs
    i) information about growth and development so that expectations of parents can be realistic
    j) assistance in learning to respond to the new baby's communication efforts (crying, facial expression, body movements)
    k) assistance in planning for continued health supervision of infant
    l) community resources available to provide assistance for parents in fulfilling their parental role

CHAPTER 22

COMPLICATIONS OCCURRING IN THE NEWBORN

I.   RESPIRATORY PROBLEMS

A.   Causes
     1. fetal anoxia prior to delivery
        a) adequate supply of oxygen to fetus is dependent upon
           (1) normal oxygenation of maternal blood
           (2) normal maternal blood pressure
           (3) adequate relaxation of uterine musculature to permit
               placental filling
           (4) adequate attachment of the placenta to the uterine
               wall
           (5) free circulation of blood through placenta and umbili-
               cal cord
           (6) no fetal circulatory abnormalities
        b) fetal anoxia is caused by
           (1) maternal conditions
               (a) hypoxia secondary to cardiac failure
               (b) hypotension as a complication of spinal anesthesia
               (c) uterine tetany from pituitrin or pitocin adminis-
                   tration
               (d) premature separation of placenta or other placen-
                   tal disturbances
               (e) placental dysfunction due to toxemia
           (2) fetal conditions
               (a) postmaturity
               (b) knotted cord
               (c) Rh factor
     2. fetal anoxia at birth
        a) may be due to predelivery influences
        b) excessive analgesia or anesthesia leading to depression
           of fetal respiratory center
        c) rapid, precipitous, prolonged or difficult delivery
        d) injury to spinal cord or phrenic nerve, especially dur-
           ing breech delivery
        e) aspiration of mucus, blood, amniotic fluid, or meconium
        f) congenital malformations compatible to intrauterine life
           but not extrauterine life
     3. neonatal anoxia
        a) obstruction of air passages
        b) congenital defects, cardiac and/or respiratory

      c) infections
        (1) bronchial pneumonia contracted in utero or shortly
           after birth, common in infants born after premature
           rupture of membranes or prolonged deliveries
      d) hemolytic diseases
      e) pre- or postmaturity
      f) respiratory distress syndrome (hyaline membrane dis-
        ease)
      g) atelectasis of lungs

B.    Classification of asphyxia neonatorum
     1. group I: infants who never breathe or those who gasp, or
       breathe irregularly or shallowly
     2. group II: vigorous hyperrespiratory effort in attempt to
       counteract hypoxia

C.    Types of anoxia
     1. anoxic anoxia is a deficit in arterial oxygen tension at which
       blood is delivered to cells
      a) hemoglobin not completely saturated
      b) occurs in hyaline membrane disease, aspiration, con-
        genital cardiac problems and cerebral defects
     2. anemic anoxia occurs when hemoglobin levels are too low
       to carry adequate oxygen to cell and oxygen intake is nor-
       mal
      a) occurs in hemolytic disorders
     3. stagnant anoxia occurs if circulation is inadequate so that
       oxygen transportation is retarded
      a) occurs in shock or hemorrhage which causes circula-
        tory collapse
     4. histotocic anoxia occurs when tissue cells are poisoned so
       that oxygen cannot be utilized
      a) occurs in poisoning from chemical or drugs, i.e., ether,
        barbiturates

D.    Major syndromes causing respiratory distress
     1. Atelectasis
      a) primary: nonexpansion of alveoli
      b) secondary: collapse occurs after initial expansion of al-
        veoli
      c) may be complete or partial
      d) symptoms.
        (1) irregular, rapid respirations
        (2) respiratory grunts, retractions, and flaring of nos-
          trils with inspiration
        (3) chest rales
        (4) skin mottled
        (5) cyanosis intermittent or constant, decreases during
          crying or oxygen therapy
        (6) diagnosed by x-ray

    e) treatment
      (1) bronchoscopy may be done
      (2) oxygen with high humidity administered
      (3) respiratory stimulants may be ordered. Examples
          of these include Nalline and Lorfan
      (4) position changed frequently to allow expansion of
          lungs
      (5) skin stimulated to induce increased respiration
      (6) antibiotics to prevent secondary infection
      (7) prevent aspiration by careful feeding
2. pneumonia
    a) aspiration pneumonia
      (1) first symptom is attack of coughing or choking
      (2) subsequent symptoms are similar to infectious pneu-
          monia
      (3) prevention
         (a) careful feeding
         (b) does not usually occur in breast-fed babies
         (c) nipple openings should not be free flowing
         (d) position baby on abdomen or side after eating
         (e) if infant chokes, it should be held upside down
           and back gently stroked to drain aspirated fluid
           from lung
    b) infectious pneumonia
      (1) cause
         (a) aspiration of infected amniotic fluid or vaginal
           secretions
         (b) contact with someone who harbors organisms
         (c) causative organisms
           1. E. coli
           2. enterococci
           3. klebsiella
           4. staphylococcus
           5. streptococcus
      (2) signs
         (a) rapid respiration
         (b) flaring of nares
         (c) respiratory grunt, retraction
         (d) temperature rises or may be subnormal
         (e) listless, pale, cyanotic
         (f) abdominal distention
         (g) refuses feeding
         (h) diagnosed by x-ray
3. neonatal respiratory distress syndrome (hyaline membrane
   disease)
    a) occurrence
      (1) prematures between 1000-1500g: the less they weigh,
          the increased incidence of RDS
      (2) babies of diabetic mothers
      (3) babies born by cesarean section

      b) caused by lack of adequate alveolar surfactant production (antiatelectasis factor) in infant lungs
         (1) lung compliance decreases and breathing becomes difficult. Alveoli collapse after each respiration. Hyperventilation and hypoperfusion of the alveoli and asphyxia may result
      c) signs
         (1) increase in respiratory rate
         (2) sternal retractions
         (3) expiratory grunt
         (4) flaring of nares
         (5) cyanosis not always apparent or may be confined to extremities
            (a) if severe, then skin appears pale and dusky
         (6) apnea spells
            (a) indicative of imminent exhaustion
         (7) gradual central nervous system depression with increasing flaccidity of musculature
      d) treatment (Behrle, 1978)
         (1) placement in a temperature environment that is not too hot or too cold, to reduce oxygen demands on tissues (neutral thermal environment)
         (2) NPO and fed by IV in early acute stage
         (3) $O_2$ administration
         (4) assisted mechanical ventilation may be needed; continuous positive airway pressure (CPAP)
         (5) monitor blood, BP and respiration
         (6) prevent acidosis
      e) complications include pulmonary hemorrhage, atelectasis, pneumothorax, sepsis
      f) infants who receive mechanical ventilation may develop bronchopulmonary dysplasia from the high $O_2$ concentrations on respiratory lining
      g) latest research indicates that administration of steroids such as dexamethasone to a mother in premature labor may stimulate the production of surfactants in the baby's lungs. Further studies must be done in this area
   4. meconium aspiration syndrome
      a) may require resuscitation at birth
      b) signs of chest retractions, tachypnea and cyanosis
      c) diagnosed by x-ray

E.    Nursing care of infants with respiratory distress
   1. assessment
      a) heart rate may be increased (over 150)
      b) temperature and skin color: cyanosis or pallor may occur; temperature may rise or fall
      c) activity and muscle tone: infant may show signs of hyperactivity or flaccidity
      d) cry: moaning or whining indicates problem

   e)  appetite may decrease or infant may have difficulty in feeding

   f)  respiration
    (1)  rate
     (a)  above 60 or rapid rise indicates danger
     (b)  increase and then decrease below 30 with periods of apnea indicates extreme danger
    (2)  rhythm
     (a)  prolonged irregularity is a danger signal
    (3)  retractions
     (a)  simple: abdomen and chest rise together with slight indentation over sternal area, flaring of nares occurs
     (b)  paradoxical: abdomen rises and chest sinks during inspiration, reversed during expiration - marked intercostal and xiphoid retraction, chin lag, respiratory grunt, and severe respiratory distress

   g)  monitor blood chemistry for signs of acidosis
   h)  check nasopharyngeal passages for presence of mucus

  2.  intervention
   a)  adequate oxygenation
   b)  maintain humidity
   c)  medications as ordered
   d)  change position frequently - cutaneous stimulation may assist in restoring respiratory pattern in apneic periods
   e)  feed carefully
   f)  gentle suction when indicated
   g)  prevent hypothermia by maintaining the temperature of the environment and by limiting infant exposure
   h)  frequent monitoring of vital signs
   i)  prevent fatigue and exhaustion
    (1)  avoid prolonged feedings
    (2)  gavage may be necessary
   j)  be prepared for periods of apnea by having oxygen apparatus ready
   k)  monitor fluid intake and output
    (1)  rate of infusions carefully controlled

## II.  BIRTH INJURIES

A.  Intracranial hemorrhage
  1.  caused by brain trauma leading to bleeding into cerebellum, pons and medulla oblongata
  2.  symptoms
   a)  cyanosis
   b)  abnormal respirations
   c)  sharp, shrill, weak cry
   d)  flaccidity
   e)  convulsions

        f) shock
        g) acidoses
    3. occurs more often in
        a) prolonged labors
        b) forceps delivery
        c) version and extraction
        d) precipitate deliveries
    4. nursing intervention
        a) effective if hemorrhage not extensive
        b) rest with minimum handling
           (1) feeding with minimum effort of infant
              (a) usually gavaged
        c) vitamins C and K to control hemorrhage as ordered
        d) head of infant kept above level of hips
        e) careful and continued observation for changes in symptoms
    5. prognosis depends on extent of damage

B.    Paralysis
    1. facial
        a) caused by pressure on facial nerve by forceps
        b) prognosis: condition transitory and usually disappears in a few days
    2. arm
        a) brachial palsy or Erb's palsy, common terms for arm paralysis
        b) caused by pressure on brachial plexus in breech extraction
        c) prognosis: recovery spontaneous within weeks or months, surgery may be needed for those few cases that do not heal spontaneously
    3. nursing intervention
        a) careful observation
        b) handle carefully to minimize trauma and discomfort
        c) for facial paralysis, careful feeding due to sucking defects
        d) parental support

C.    Fractures and dislocations
    1. most commonly seen in version or breech deliveries
    2. fractures are common in long bones, clavicle or jaw
    3. fractures heal rapidly
    4. fractures need immobilization
    5. dislocations must be reduced immediately

III.    HEMOLYTIC DISEASE OF NEWBORN

A.    ABO incompatibility
    1. mild hemolytic disease
    2. father's blood type is A or B, mother's blood type is O, baby will therefore be type A or B

    3. baby produces A or B antigens which enter mother's bloodstream, causing mother to produce A or B antibodies. These antibodies cross back into baby's bloodstream and cause hemolysis of baby's red blood cells

    4. symptoms
       a) jaundice occurring within 48 hours
       b) mild anemia
       c) negative or low Coombs' test

    5. treatment
       a) light therapy
         (1) undressed baby is exposed to fluorescent daylight bulbs, eyes are covered
         (2) bilirubin is decomposed by photo-oxidation in the skin
       b) exchange transfusion if bilirubin rises above 20 mg/100 ml of blood
       c) prognosis: usually recovers spontaneously

B.    Rh incompatibility

    1. when mother is Rh-negative and father is Rh-positive, the mother's blood does not contain the Rh factor whereas it is present in the father's. Since the Rh factor is a dominant gene there is a high probability that the baby will be Rh-positive. At the birth of the first Rh-positive baby, the Rh factor may enter the mother's bloodstream causing her to form antibodies to this factor. In subsequent pregnancies these maternal antibodies may cross the placental barrier and enter the fetal bloodstream. This may cause hemolysis of the red blood cells if the baby is Rh-positive. Sensitization of the mother may also occur if she has received a Rh-positive blood transfusion

    2. RhoGAM is a vaccine that must be used within 72 hours after delivery to prevent sensitization of mother to the Rh-positive factor

    3. erythroblastosis fetalis: is the condition of the infant which occurs because of Rh incompatibility: incidence has greatly diminished because of use of RhoGAM
       a) signs and symptoms
         (1) anemia present at birth or soon after, varies in severity
         (2) vernix caseosa yellow
         (3) jaundice occurring within 24 hours
         (4) enlarged liver and spleen
         (5) positive Coombs' test
         (6) elevates serum bilirubin
       b) hydrops fetalis
         (1) most severe form of erythroblastosis fetalis
         (2) symptoms
           (a) generalized edema of the infant beginning in utero
           (b) marked anemia
           (c) severe jaundice
           (d) enlarged liver and spleen

        (3) prognosis
           (a) infant usually stillborn
           (b) if born alive invariably dies within short period
     c) kernicterus
        (1) occurs when central nervous system becomes involved due to persistent high bilirubin levels (20 mg/ 100 ml of blood)
        (2) symptoms
           (a) anorexia
           (b) lethargy
           (c) abnormal Moro reflex
           (d) opisthotonos
           (e) convulsions
           (f) spasticity
        (3) prognosis
           (a) high death rate
           (b) mental retardation
  4. treatment of Rh incompatibility
     a) prevented by use of RhoGAM
     b) careful check of antibody titer levels in mother during pregnancy
     c) if titer levels are high or increase rapidly, intrauterine exchange transfusion may be done
     d) fresh Rh-negative blood is used for transfusion
     e) Coombs' test done at birth from cord blood
     f) careful monitoring of bilirubin level
     g) exchange transfusion if bilirubin level remains high
     h) light therapy

C.  Nursing implications:  hemolytic disease of the newborn
  1. assessment
     a) check for early signs and symptoms relating to the manifestations of hemolytic disease
     b) continuing assessment for any worsening of symptoms
     c) observe for reactions to phototherapy
  2. intervention
     a) phototherapy
        (1) protect eyes during therapy
        (2) remove eye protection during feeding and bathing to provide sensory stimulation

IV.  INFECTIONS

A.  Neonate has lower resistance to pathogens because antibodies are not developed
  1. most common bacterial and viral pathogens causing infection
     a) staphylococcus aureus
        (1) causes respiratory infection and impetigo

      b) staphylococcus coagulase positive (hospital staph) is resistant to most antibiotics; causes impetigo and infection in any open skin tissue

      c) streptococcus causes skin and respiratory infections

      d) <u>E. coli</u> causes respiratory and gastrointestinal infections

      e) salmonella causes respiratory and gastrointestinal infections

      f) shigella causes respiratory and gastrointestinal infections

      g) viruses cause gastrointestinal and respiratory infections

2. modes of transmission

      a) through nose and throat secretions of nursery personnel and mother

      b) skin infection of personnel and mother

      c) poor hand washing technique

      d) fomite contamination

         (1) humidifiers

         (2) faucets

         (3) sinks

         (4) articles of infant care

3. disease manifestations of pathogens

      a) impetigo

      b) respiratory infections

      c) cord infections

      d) circumcision infections

      e) gastrointestinal disturbance

         (1) diarrhea

         (2) vomiting

      f) eye infections

      g) septicemia

B. Ophthalmia neonatorum

1. infection of eye caused by gonococcus and chlamydial organisms

2. acquired during delivery from mother's vaginal canal

3. may result in blindness if not treated

4. state law requires preventive treatment

      a) silver nitrate 1% (effective only for GC)

      b) antibiotic eye ointment (effective for both organisms)

C. Thrush is an infectious disease of the newborn caused by <u>Candida Albicans</u> which is a fungus

1. transmission

      a) acquired during delivery if mother has a monilia infection

      b) acquired from infected personnel who use poor aseptic

2. symptoms include mucus white patches on mucosa of mouth that cannot be removed

3. treatment

        a) antibiotics
        b) gentian violet 1% applied to lesion

D.    Congenital syphilis
        1. preventable by treatment in early pregnancy
        2. symptoms may be present at birth or may occur up to 4
           months of age
            a) highly infectious skin lesions found primarily on
                (1) face
                (2) buttocks
                (3) palms
                (4) soles of feet
            b) mucus patches
                (1) mouth
                (2) anus
            c) rhinitis (snuffles)
            d) hoarseness
            e) deformity of nails
            f) alopecia
            g) enlargement of lymph nodes
            h) enlargement of liver and spleen
            i) osteochondritis of long bones
            j) central nervous system involvement
        3. diagnosis made from symptoms with a positive serology
        4. treatment
            a) isolation
            b) antibiotics

E.    Acute necrotizing enterocolitis
        1. predisposing factors include prematurity, RDA, apneic
           spells, or other severe perinatal stressors
        2. symptoms
            a) vomiting (bile and blood)
            b) lethargic, poor appetite
            c) abdominal distention
        3. causes include early feeding of prematures with formula,
           injury to intestinal mucosa, and bacterial infection
        4. condition may be mild or severe.  In severe cases there is
           a high mortality rate
        5. treatment
            a) antibiotics
            b) NPO
            c) IV fluids
        6. human breast milk may play an important role in prevent-
           ing this condition

F.    Epidemic diarrhea
        1. causes
            a) staphylococcus
            b) E. coli most common organisms

        c) predisposing factors
          (1) overcrowding in nursery
          (2) poor personal hygiene of personnel and mothers
          (3) poor aseptic nursery technique
    2. symptoms: sudden onset of profuse watery stools
    3. treatment
        a) immediate isolation
        b) antibiotics
        c) prevention of dehydration through use of intravenous feeding
    4. prognosis: high mortality rate

G.    Nursing implication in infections of newborn
    1. assessment
        a) monitoring of vital signs
          (1) in many cases during an infectious process there may not be a rise in temperature
        b) observe for signs of infection
          (1) lethargy
          (2) anorexia
          (3) irritability
          (4) abnormal discharge from body orifices
          (5) skin eruptions or inflammation
          (6) abnormal bowel or bladder manifestations
          (7) respiratory irregularities
          (8) changes in skin color
          (9) mucous membrane lesions
    2. intervention
        a) immediate isolation of infected baby and personnel
        b) aseptic technique carefully followed
        c) treatment of infection with appropriate drugs
        d) prevention of complication, i.e., dehydration
        e) support, information and reassurance to parents

V.    CONGENITAL ANOMALIES

A.    Classification
    1. anomalies compatible with intrauterine life only (i.e., anencephaly)
    2. anomalies compatible with extrauterine life, only with immediate surgical intervention (i.e., imperforate anus)
    3. anomalies compatible with extrauterine life (i.e., umbilical hernia)

B.    CNS abnormalities
    1. anencephaly is a malformation of the brain and/or cerebral hemispheres. Scalp and cranium may be missing
        a) prognosis: no chance of survival
    2. hydrocephalus: CSF is not absorbed from intracranial cavity. Normal circulation of fluid may be disturbed because

of obstruction. May have excess secretion of fluid or there may be an absorption problem

    a) prognosis: condition is not fatal. Secondary causes may lead to death. Mental retardation may occur if untreated

    b) treatment

        (1) shunts may be used to alleviate excessive fluid

        (2) shunts may have to be repeated (40%)

        (3) complications of shunts include septicemia and pulmonary thromboses

3. spina bifida is a defect in closure of spinal column. Membranes surrounding the spinal cord, and/or the spinal cord may protrude from opening. It is called meningocele or myomeningocele and is often accompanied by hydrocephalus

    a) prognosis is poor, child is usually paraplegic

    b) treatment

        (1) closure of spinal column

        (2) rehabilitative treatment

4. nursing implications

    a) assessment

        (1) observe for abnormalities in reflex reactions

        (2) accurate measurements of head

        (3) signs of irritability, lethargy, twitching and tremors

        (4) frequency and length of convulsions

        (5) skin condition around myomeningocele

        (6) feeding behavior

        (7) skin breakdown in case of hydrocephalus

        (8) changes in vital signs

    b) intervention

        (1) change position frequently

        (2) protect baby from injury during convulsions

        (3) reduce irritating stimuli such as noise or sudden movements to decrease incidence of convulsions

        (4) careful feeding practices

        (5) use padding to prevent pressure near and around abnormalities

C.    Congenital heart disease (more deaths occur from CHD than any other anomaly)

    1. patent ductus is a fetal opening between pulmonary artery and aorta which fails to close at birth

        a) corrected by surgery with good prognosis

    2. patent foramen ovale is a fetal opening between right and left atrium which fails to close at birth

        a) corrected by surgery with good results

    3. ventricular septal defects

        a) vary in size

        b) blood shunts from right to left ventricle

      c) if defect is small, no treatment is necessary and may close normally. Large defects require surgery

  4. coarctation of the aorta (stenosis)
      a) narrowing of aorta
      b) may be corrected by surgery with good prognosis

  5. tetralogy of Fallot
      a) combination of four defects
         (1) pulmonary stenosis
         (2) ventricular septal defect
         (3) overriding aorta
         (4) hypertrophy of right ventricle
      b) can be corrected by surgery, mortality rate high

  6. transposition of the great vessels
      a) vessels arise out of the wrong ventricles
      b) corrected by surgery with a high mortality rate

  7. other defects occur rarely

  8. symptoms of newborns with congenital heart disease
      a) cyanosis
      b) dyspnea
      c) tachycardia
      d) difficulty with feeding
      e) failure to thrive
      f) heart murmurs
      g) stridor or choking spells
      h) anoxic attacks

  9. surgery is usually performed very early

D.    Respiratory system
  1. congenital laryngeal stridor
      a) abnormality in or around larynx
      b) symptoms
         (1) noisy respiration
         (2) crowing sound in inspiration
      c) surgery indicated if condition is severe

  2. occlusion of nasal passage
      a) may be either unilateral or bilateral
      b) usually obstructed at junction of nasopharynx by membrane or bony growth
      c) symptoms
         (1) dyspnea
         (2) difficulty in feeding
         (3) mouth breathing
      d) treated by surgical intervention

E.    Nursing implications in abnormalities of respiratory system and congenital heart disease
  1. assessment
      a) vital signs
      b) color
      c) dyspnea and abnormal respiratory patterns
      d) character of cry

        e)  effect of crying on physiological status
        f)  feeding behavior
        g)  nutritional status
        h)  intake and output
  2. intervention
        a)  maintain patent airway
        b)  careful monitoring of oxygen therapy
        c)  careful slow feeding
        d)  avoid fatiguing infant
        e)  change position frequently
        f)  continuing observation is vital to detect periods of apnea

F.    Gastrointestinal malformations
  1. tongue tie: frenum linguae
        a)  vertical fold of mucous membrane under tongue some-
            times interferes with sucking and speech
        b)  can be corrected surgically
  2. cleft lip and cleft palate
        a)  failure of maxillary and palatal processes to close
        b)  leads to problems in feeding, speech and danger of infec-
            tion
        c)  corrected surgically
        d)  speech therapy when older
  3. esophageal atresia
        a)  absence of closure of esophagus
            (1)  during feeding, chokes and turns blue
            (2)  excessive drooling and mucus secretion
            (3)  corrected by surgery
  4. tracheoesophageal fistula
        a)  opening between trachea and esophagus
        b)  symptoms and treatment same as esophageal atresia
  5. pyloric stenosis
        a)  hypertrophy of pyloric muscles interfere with emptying
            contents of stomach
        b)  symptoms include projectile vomiting after feeding
        c)  corrected by surgery with good prognosis
  6. intestinal obstructions
        a)  complete or partial by stenosis or atresia at any level
            of intestinal tract
        b)  vomiting and no stools are prime symptoms
        c)  corrected by surgery
  7. imperforate anus
        a)  membrane over anal opening or absence of anus
        b)  no stools
        c)  surgery to correct
  8. biliary tract obstruction
        a)  flow of bile into intestine is blocked
        b)  symptoms include clay color or white stools, jaundiced,
            bile stained urine
        c)  corrected by surgery

9. omphalocele
   a) intestine protrudes out of umbilicus without skin covering
   b) must be protected with wet dressing until surgery
   c) surgery to correct
10. umbilical hernia
    a) protrusion of intestine with skin covering at umbilicus
    b) may reduce spontaneously without surgery
11. nursing implications in gastrointestinal malformations
    a) assessment
       (1) feeding behavior
       (2) presence, time of occurrence, frequency and character of vomiting
       (3) bowel function: character and frequency of stools
       (4) excess salivation and drooling
       (5) nutritional status
       (6) structure of mouth
       (7) patency of rectum
       (8) check condition of umbilical cord stump
    b) intervention
       (1) careful and appropriate feeding to prevent aspiration
       (2) maintain fluid intake

G. Genitourinary system
   1. hypospadias: urethra opens on lower surface of penis, can be corrected by surgery
   2. agenesis of kidneys or ureters incompatible with extrauterine life
   3. cystic or polycystic kidneys can in later life interfere with urine production
   4. extrophy of bladder is a partial or complete exposure of bladder through abdominal wall

H. Musculoskeletal system
   1. clubfoot: talipes equinovarus
      a) adduction and supination of forefoot
      b) may be casted or placed in Dennis and Brown splint
   2. congenital dislocation of hip
      a) head of femur not in acetabulum
      b) placed in cast
   3. torticollis (wryneck)
      a) head in downward position on one side with chin rotated to the other side
      b) corrected by exercise
      c) two-thirds disappear with little or no treatment
      d) if persistent or recurrent, resection of muscles is necessary

VI.   INBORN ERRORS OF METABOLISM

A.   Phenylketonuria (PKU)
   1. enzyme necessary to break down phenylalanine is absent
   2. phenylalanine builds up in brain causing mental retardation
   3. early detection is possible because of mandatory blood testing of newborns in many states
   4. mental retardation can be prevented by a diet which excludes phenylalanine

B.   Other syndromes include galactosemia and maple sugar urine disease

VII.   CHROMOSOMAL ABERRATIONS

A.   Down's syndrome (trisomy 21)
   1. child has 47 chromosomes
   2. characteristics
     a) slanting eyes
     b) flat nose
     c) simian palm crease
     d) wide space between second and third toes
     e) protruding tongue
     f) broad, pudgy neck
     g) muscles flaccid
   3. mental retardation may range from moderate to profound
   4. very often other congenital defects are also present

B.   Other syndromes include Klinefelter's and Turner's which are caused by extra sex chromosomes

VIII.   BABY OF A DIABETIC MOTHER

A.   Effect of diabetes in mother on fetus
   1. glucose crosses placenta and insulin does not, causing increased blood sugar levels in fetus
   2. fetus reacts by increasing his output of insulin
   3. increased insulin production may lead to hypertrophy of pancreas
   4. increased danger of stillbirth

B.   Effect of diabetic mother on infant
   1. hyperinsulin production may occur leading to hypoglycemia
   2. over-sized baby who may be immature
   3. increased incidence of respiratory distress syndrome
   4. increased incidence of congenital malformations
   5. hypocalcemia or hypomagnesemia may occur
   6. hyperbilirubinemia during first 42-72 hours of life may occur

C. Treatment
1. careful control of mother's diabetic status through insulin, diet and activity regulation
2. early delivery through induction or cesarean section
3. maintain infant's fluid and electrolyte balance to prevent acidosis
4. hourly blood glucose monitoring for 4-6 hours after birth. If hypoglycemia occurs, IV glucose is given
5. phototherapy may be needed in high bilirubin levels

D. Nursing implications
1. assessment of infant for
   a) irritability, tremors, twitches and convulsions may indicate hypocalcemia
   b) blood chemistry deviations
   c) neurological assessment
   d) vital signs
   e) intake and output
   f) vomiting or diarrhea which may influence fluid and electrolyte balance
   g) feeding behavior
   h) nutritional status
2. intervention
   a) monitor parental therapy to prevent injury and rapid overhydration
   b) report any significant changes in fluid and electrolyte balance and neurological status
   c) careful positioning to decrease respiratory difficulties
   d) careful feeding
   e) treated as if premature

IX. POSTMATURITY

A. Pregnancy that exceeds 42 or 43 weeks

B. Oversize fetus may cause problems in labor and delivery

C. Not all prolonged pregnancies are postmature as the EDC is not always accurate

D. An accurate gestational age must be determined through sonogram and fundal measurements

E. Fetal status is monitored through 24-hour urinary estrial, maternal plasma HCS levels, and oxytocin challenge tests

F. If fetal state is normal, pregnancy is allowed to go to term

G. If fetal distress or dysmaturity is found, labor is induced

H. Physical signs of post-term infants include desquamation of skin, long fingernails, and meconium staining of skin

X.  PARENTAL REACTION TO THE NEWBORN WITH COMPLI-
    CATIONS

A.  Parents go through grieving process which may include
    1. hostility to staff
    2. guilt feelings about their responsibility for defect
    3. denial
    4. rejection of child

B.  Should be educated to understand causes of defects during
    prenatal period

C.  Opportunity after delivery to ventilate feelings and grief
    should be offered

D.  Need early contact with and responsibility for care of child

E.  Need continuous support and understanding by health profes-
    sional

# CHAPTER 23

# THE PRETERM AND LOW BIRTH WEIGHT INFANT

I. DEFINITION

A. Premature: born before 37 weeks gestation; also known as preterm infants

B. Low birth weight infant: weight is below tenth percentile for gestational age also known as small for gestational age baby (SGA)

II. ETIOLOGY

A. Is not known but contributing factors include
   1. poor nutrition
   2. poor living conditions
   3. fatigue due to overwork
   4. poor health habits
   5. multiple births
   6. preeclampsia
   7. antepartal hemorrhage
   8. premature rupture of membranes
   9. hydramnios
   10. trauma
   11. chronic or acute infection or disease in mother
   12. emotional stress
   13. congenital fetal malformation
   14. endocrine disturbances
   15. smoking
   16. placental abnormalities
   17. maternal age under 19
   18. anemia

III. DIAGNOSIS OF IUGR (INTRAUTERINE GROWTH RETARDATION)

A. Slow increase in fundal height measurements

B. Low or decreasing 24-hour urinary estrogens

C. Lack of adequate growth in fetal biparietal diameter (ultrasound scanning)

IV. PREVENTION

A. Prevention of preterm births
   1. early and regular prenatal care
   2. cessation of smoking
   3. surgical intervention for incompetent cervix (purse-string surgery)
   4. prolongation of the pregnancy through
      a) bed rest
      b) ethanol therapy
      c) the use of beta-adrenergic drugs are under investigation
   5. adequate nutrition
   6. reduce stress

B. Prevention of IUGR
   1. treatment or prevention of associated causes
   2. monitoring of fetal growth and status
   3. improvement of maternal nutrition
   4. bed rest
   5. delivery timed to prevent fetal distress while ensuring an optimum level of development in some instances of IUGR

V. STATISTICAL FACTS

A. 5-8% of total newborns are preterm

B. 2-10% of newborns are SGA

C. Survival rates for infants over 1000 g are good if expert care is provided

D. Higher incidences of CNS handicaps in infants whose birth weight is less than 1500 g

E. Increased perinatal morbidity, mortality, and congenital abnormalities

VI. PHYSICAL CHARACTERISTICS OF PRETERM INFANT

A. The characteristics will vary with gestational age and weight
   1. determining whether the newborn is preterm rather than SGA, the following physical screening devices to determine gestational age are useful
      a) sole creases
         (1) preterm infant: has few or no sole creases
         (2) full term infant: has more and deeper creases
      b) ears
         (1) preterm: flat and shapeless
         (2) mature infant: has incurving of 2/3 of pinna
      c) breast
         (1) preterm: the nipples are hard to detect and no breast tissue

(2) mature infant: has a raised areola and a small amount of breast tissue
- d) genitals
  - (1) male
    - (a) preterm: testes are high in canal, few ruggae are present in scrotum
    - (b) full term: testes are lower and many ruggae are present
  - (2) female
    - (a) preterm: clitoris prominent and labia majora are small
    - (b) full term: labia majora covers the clitoris
2. additional observations of physical and neurological signs may also be done

B. Color
1. pink or dark red
2. acrocyanosis
3. cyanotic
4. jaundiced

C. Cry
1. feeble
2. cries infrequently

D. Activity
1. usually reduced
2. poor muscle tone

E. Reflexes
1. sucking, gagging, and swallowing may be absent or feeble
2. tonic neck and Moro may be present or ill-defined

F. Skin
1. small amount of vernix caseosa
2. ecchymotic areas common
3. large amounts of lanugo
4. little if any subcutaneous fat

G. Head and face
1. large in proportion to body size
2. fontanels small
3. head round or ovoid with little molding
4. features sharp and angular

H. Chest
1. thoracic rib cage weak due to immature bone calcification

I. Genitalia
1. enlarged labia minora and clitoris
2. testes may be undescended

VII. PROBLEMS OF PRETERM INFANTS AND SGA INFANTS

A. Respiratory
1. caused by
a) immature chest, muscular and skeletal development
b) weak gag and cough reflexes
2. lead to danger of
a) atelectasis
b) apnea
c) respiratory infections
d) respiratory distress syndrome

B. Feeding problems
1. caused by
a) weak sucking and swallowing reflexes
b) small stomach capacity
2. may lead to
a) aspiration
b) inadequate intake
c) abdominal distention
d) vomiting

C. Problem of maintaining body temperature
1. caused by
a) excessive loss of heat by radiation
b) lack of heat production due to inactivity
c) small amount of subcutaneous fat
d) skin capillaries not well controlled

D. Problem of unstable acid-base and electrolytic balance
1. caused by renal immaturity
2. may lead to
a) edema
b) acidosis
c) dehydration
d) oliguria

E. Problem of hemolytic immaturity
1. caused by
a) capillary fragility and permeability
b) inability to synthesize vitamin K
c) immature liver functioning
2. may lead to
a) jaundice
b) petechiae
c) ecchymosis
d) hemorrhage

F. Resistance to infection reduced because of
1. reduced immune substances from mother due to inability to breast feed and lack of placental transmission of antibodies which occurs in last trimester

2. immaturity of homeostatic responses

G. Problems of CNS
   1. caused by
      a) immaturity of CNS
      b) anoxia
      c) prolonged prothrombin time leading to intracranial hemorrhage

H. Persistent patent ductus arteriosus may lead to congestive heart failure

VIII. NURSING IMPLICATIONS

A. Assessment
   1. respirations
      a) rate and quality
      b) dyspnea, apnea, or tachypnea
         (1) tachypnea: respirations over 60/min
         (2) may be a sign of complication such as anemia, CNS problem, RDS
         (3) may be due to high environmental temperature or transitory tachypnea of the newborn which disappears spontaneously in 2-3 days
      c) sternal and costal retractions
      d) nasal flaring
      e) cyanosis
   2. temperature
   3. heart rate
   4. reflexes
   5. neurological symptoms (tremors, twitching, convulsions, irritability, lethargy)
   6. intake and output
      a) check for signs of dehydration including poor skin turgor, lethargy, lowered urinary output, loss of weight, dry skin
   7. skin, turgor, color and condition
   8. edema
   9. change in activity
   10. blood gases
   11. blood chemistries
   12. sucking ability
   13. feeding behavior
   14. cry
   15. muscle tone
   16. reaction to stimuli
   17. presence of petechiae, ecchymosis
   18. abdominal distention
   19. frequency, amount and character of stools and urine
   20. vomiting
   21. weight gain

B.  Intervention
    1. maintain body temperature
       a) neonatal heat loss occurs through radiation, conduction, convection and evaporation. After birth the neonate loses heat by radiation to cold wall of delivery room or isolette or if placed on a metal table or through moving air currents
       b) the mature infant can increase heat production through nonshivering thermogenesis. The premature infant has less ability to do this
       c) when the premature suffers heat loss he may develop acidosis, hypoxia and hypoglycemia
       d) newborn should be dryed immediately, placed under radiant heat, wrapped in warm blankets or placed in warm incubator. Oxygen should be warmed and humidified
       e) abdominal skin temperature should be kept at 97-98°F
       f) hyperthermia should be avoided
    2. oxygen and humidity in isolette should be maintained
       a) oxygen tension of arterial blood should not exceed 100 mm Hg and should be maintained between 60-80 mm Hg
       b) if child develops cyanosis at the maximum level of oxygen intake prescribed to prevent retrolental fibroplasia (40% concentration) then a higher concentration of oxygen may be necessary. This can only be administered under conditions where continuous monitoring of blood gases is possible
       c) concentration of oxygen must be analyzed every two hours with an oxygen analyzer. Performance of analyzer must be checked daily
       d) neonate must be observed for periods of dyspnea and apnea. Apnea is particularly likely to occur during REM sleep. Management of apnea includes treating underlying cause if there is one and also the apnea itself. Stroking of the skin is helpful; bag and mask resuscitation may be needed
    3. feeding: intake should be 100/120 cal/ng of body weight
       a) if sucking reflex is absent gavage or parental feeding may be administered
          (1) if gavage is necessary always lubricate tube with water rather than oil
          (2) chill tube to facilitate insertion
          (3) check placement of tube in stomach through aspiration of stomach contents by negative pressure from a syringe
          (4) slow feeding with constant observation
       b) gavage and IV fluids are also used if the sucking reflex is intermittent
       c) complications of gavage include vagal stimulation with apnea and bradycardia
       d) check for regurgitation, cyanosis, respiratory problems, abdominal distention when using intermittent gavage or indwelling nasal catheter

       e) slow, small frequent feedings if sucking reflex is present
       f) place on side after feeding to prevent aspiration
       g) if parental fluid is administered monitor drip rate carefully to prevent overhydration
       h) assure adequate intake of nutrients

    4. positioning
       a) change position frequently
       b) handle gently and carefully to prevent injury
       c) maintain normal body alignment

    5. aseptic technique to prevent infections
    6. sensory stimulation
       a) recent research indicates that prematures may benefit from increased and early auditory, visual and tactile and kinesthetic stimulation

## IX. PARENT'S NEEDS

A.    May feel guilt and anxiety: may be afraid to touch or handle infant

B.    Instruction regarding care of infant

C.    Reassurance and support: encourage ventilation of feelings

D.    As early as possible, parents should assume responsibility for care of child to encourage bonding

E.    Follow-up referral for nursing supervision on discharge

## STUDY QUESTIONS

1. What predisposing factors may lead to fetal anoxia?
2. What signs and symptoms indicate the presence of fetal anoxia?
3. What is the treatment of fetal anoxia?
4. What conditions may interfere with normal feeding process in the newborn?
5. What is the significance of a weight loss in the first week of life?
6. What is the difference between jaundice occurring in first 12 hours and jaundice occurring on third day of life?
7. Differentiate between stools of breast-fed and bottle-fed baby after fifth day of life.
8. What are the disadvantages of physiological resilience?
9. What symptoms in the newborn may indicate pathology?
10. How is infection of the newborn controlled in the nursery?
11. What conditions may occur in the newborn as a result of a difficult labor?
12. What is the nursing care for a baby who has been circumcised?
13. Bulging of the fontanels has what meaning?
14. What are the clinical manifestations of the infant who has erythroblastosis fetalis?

15. A decision to use an exchange transfusion in an infant with erythroblastosis fetalis is dependent on which laboratory tests?
16. What condition in an infant is associated with projectile vomiting?
17. What precautions should be taken when feeding an infant with a cleft palate?
18. Define the term prematurity in terms of weight classification?
19. What is the relationship between the weight of the premature and its prognosis?
20. What physiological handicaps are overcome by placing a premature infant in an incubator?
21. What is the danger of a "high oxygen concentration" in the incubator?
22. What are the symptoms and the treatment of respiratory distress syndrome?

## BIBLIOGRAPHY

Alden, E.R., Mandelkorn, T., et al.: Morbidity and Mortality of Infants Weighing Less Than 1000 g in an Intensive Care Nursery, Pediatrics 50:40, 1972.

Arnold, Helen, et al.: The Newborn, Transition to Extrauterine Life, American Journal of Nursing, October, 1965.

Barson, C., et al.: Neonatal Diabetes, Nursing Mirror, March 29, 1974.

Bash, B.D. and Gold, A.W.: The Nurse and the Childbearing Family, John Wiley, N.Y., 1981, pp. 584-588.

Behrle, F.: Respiratory Distress Syndrome, in: Perinatology Case Studies (L. Iffy and A. Langer, eds.), Med. Exam. Publ. Co., Garden City, N.Y., 1978, pp. 481-491.

Brazelton, J.B.: Neonatal Behavioral Assessment Scale, in: Clinics in Developmental Medicine, #50, J.B. Lippincott, Philadelphia, 1973, pp. 7-9.

Bruce, S.: Reactions of Nurses and Mothers to Stillbirths, Nursing Outlook, February, 1962.

Chinn, Peggy: Infant Gavage Feeding, American Journal of Nursing, October, 1971.

Diller, L: Psychology of Disabled Children, American Journal of Nursing, July, 1964.

Engel, G.L.: Grief and Grieving, American Journal of Nursing, September, 1964.

Fleming, J.W.: Recognizing the Newborn Addict, American Journal of Nursing, January, 1965.

Frank, L.: On the Importance of Infancy, Random House, N.Y., 1968.

Gillon, J.E.: Behavior of Newborns with Cardiac Distress, American Journal of Nursing, February, 1973.

Glista, B.: Problems of the Very Premature Newborn, in: Perinatology Case Studies (L. Iffy and A. Langer, eds.), Med. Exam. Publ. Co., Garden City, N.Y., 1978, pp. 541-543.

Haynes, Una: A Developmental Approach to Casefinding, U.S. Dept. H.E.W., Childrens Bureau, 1967.

Justice, P., et al.: Phenylketonuria, American Journal of Nursing, August, 1975.

Klaus, M.H. and Kennell, J.H.: Care of the High-Risk Neonate, St. Louis, C.V. Mosby Co., 1976.

Korones, S., et al.: High Risk Newborn Infants, St. Louis, C.V. Mosby Co., 1972.

McLenehan, I.G.: No Baby to Take Home, American Journal of Nursing, April, 1962.

Mercer, R.T.: Mothers' Responses to their Infants with Defects, Nursing Research, March, April, 1974.

Owens, O.: Parent's Reactions to Defective Babies, American Journal of Nursing, August, 1960.

Ribble, Margaret: The Rights of Infants, Columbia University Press, N.Y., 1966.

Rhymes, Julina, P.: Working with Mothers and Babies Who Fail to Thrive, American Journal of Nursing, September, 1966.

Schultze, F.J.: Apnea, Clinics in Perinatology 4:65, 1977.

Shapiro, C.S., et al.: Nursing Care of the Cleft Lip/Cleft Palate Child, RN, August, 1973.

Warrick, L.H.: Family-Centered Care in the Premature Nursery, American Journal of Nursing, November, 1971.

# APPENDIX

## LABORATORY TESTS USED TO
## IDENTIFY FETUSES AT RISK

A.  Estriol Determinations

1. Estriol is the predominant estrogen produced during pregnancy
2. Serial determinations can assist in assessing fetal status in hypertension, diabetes, placental insufficiency states, and other conditions
3. Significant fall in urinary estriol is 35%
4. Significant fall in plasma estriol is 50%
5. Signs of fetal distress include a downward trend or precipitous fall
6. False negative results are rare
7. False positive results occur about 1/3 of cases
8. In interpreting estriol values, factors such as maternal renal disease, drugs, multiple pregnancies, bed rest and other conditions which may increase or decrease estriol levels, must be considered
9. Values for estriol should be taken serially and compared to earlier values because of the wide range of normal values

B.  L/S Ratio

1. Measures surfactant activity of fetal lung by assessing amniotic fluid
2. A value of 1.5-1 indicates an immature lung with a risk of RDS
3. A value of 2.0 indicates a mature lung with low risk of RDS except for an infant of a diabetic mother

C.  Stress Test - OCT - Oxytocin Challenge Test - Tests placental function

1. Observation of fetal heart rate in response to natural or oxytocin induced uterine contractions
2. Contractions decrease flow of oxygenated blood to fetus
3. When there is placental insufficiency the fetus will respond with heart rate deceleration

      4. At least three contractions must occur within a ten-minute period
      5. Negative test – no late deceleration (slowing of heart-rate at peak of contraction)
      6. Positive – late deceleration occurs with most contractions
      7. Rate of false positives is fairly high ( a false positive is when the late decelerations occur during the OCT but not during labor)

C.    Non Stress Test

      1. Baseline variations and accelerations of the FHR during fetal movements are observed with fetal monitoring
      2. Normal variability is usually 10 beat/min
      3. Loss of variability may result from a hypoxic condition of fetus
      4. A nonreactive non-stress test should be followed by an OCT

D.    Ultrasonography

      1. Used to establish gestational age and monitor fetal growth
      2. Diagnose multiple pregnancies
      3. Locate placenta – detect abnormalities
      4. Detection of congenital anomalies

E.    Amniotic Fluid Analyses

      1. Cell karyotypes
      2. Bilirubin values
      3. L/S ratio
      4. Neural tube defects
      5. Other congenital anomalies

# INDEX